The
Oil Pulling
Miracle

Detoxify Simply and Effectively

Birgit Frohn

Translated by Aida Sefic Williams
with assistance from John R. Baker

Healing Arts Press
Rochester, Vermont • Toronto, Canada

Healing Arts Press
One Park Street
Rochester, Vermont 05767
www.HealingArtsPress.com

Healing Arts Press is a division of Inner Traditions International

Originally published in German under the title *Die Ölzieh-Kur: Einfach und wirksam entgiften* by Mankau Verlag GmbH
First U.S. edition published in 2016 by Healing Arts Press

Note to the reader: This book is intended as an informational guide. The remedies, approaches, and techniques described herein are meant to supplement, and not to be a substitute for, professional medical care or treatment. They should not be used to treat a serious ailment without prior consultation with a qualified health care professional.

Library of Congress Cataloging-in-Publication Data
Frohn, Birgit, 1967-
  [Olzieh-Kur. English]
  The oil pulling miracle : detoxify simply and effectively / Birgit Frohn ; translated by Aida Sefic Williams.
       pages cm
  Includes bibliographical references and index.
  ISBN 978-1-62055-327-5 (paperback) — ISBN 978-1-62055-328-2 (e-book)
  1. Detoxification (Health) 2. Vegetable oils—Therapeutic use.
  3. Mouth—Care and hygiene. 4. Materia medica. I. Title.
  RA784.5.F76 2016
  613.2—dc23

                                                              2015009206

Printed and bound in the United States by Versa Press, Inc.

10 9 8 7 6 5 4 3 2 1

Text design by Priscilla Baker and layout by Debbie Glogover
This book was typeset in Garamond Premier Pro with Helvetica Neue, Gill Sans, and Cantoria for display fonts.
See page 122 for image credits.

Contents

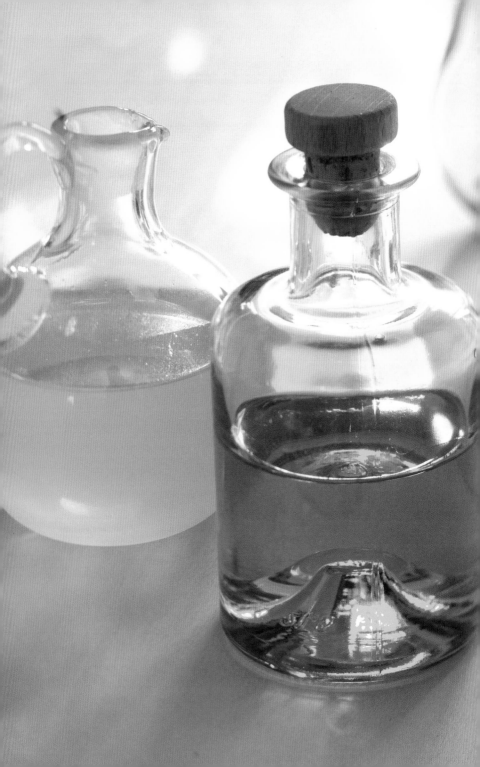

The Long Tradition
of Oil Pulling

The practice of oil pulling can be traced back for over a thousand years. That this practice has such a long tradition should come as no surprise, for the insight that our body must be regularly cleansed of waste products and toxins to maintain our health is not new. Certainly, various methods of purifying and detoxifying the body have played an enduring role in the treatment regimens of many branches of the healing arts, in many cultures, since the beginning of medicine.

The purpose of this book is to introduce you to the practice of oil pulling and to provide tips and guidelines for its use. As well, there are a variety of other detoxification techniques that beautifully complement oil pulling that we shall touch on later in this book. To stay healthy, our body requires cleansing from the inside as well as the outside. As already noted, this is not a modern insight. Long ago, the physicians of ancient Egypt prescribed special therapies designed to purify the body of toxins. Some of these involved laxatives, while others consisted of herbal preparations for internal consumption to bring about specific cleansing effects in the organs. Oil pulling, too, found a way into the repertoire of the great ancient medical traditions. Because oil pulling was regarded as a comprehensively effective method for purifying and detoxifying, it was only natural that it would be incorporated into the materia medica of those classical systems of healing.

It may surprise a few people to know that the roots of our modern Western medical system reach all the way back to India, China, and the ancient cultures of the Mediterranean region. The founding fathers of these ancient systems of medicine include the scholar Charaka and the surgeon Sushruta, both of whom helped establish the ayurvedic tradition of India; the Yellow Emperor, Huangdi, the legendary founder of traditional Chinese medicine; and Hippocrates, who along with his students established the healing traditions of the ancient Greeks, on which much of our current medical model in the West is based.

Ayurveda—the Mother of Medicine and Oil Pulling

An ideal medicine not only heals illness; it provides effective, long-lasting prevention of getting sick in the first place. On this point, all of the Asian medical traditions agree. This is the reason why these ancient healing traditions continue to advocate the use of detoxifying and purifying regimens for maintaining health and well-being. Many of these resemble the practices of ayurveda, the traditional medicine of India, in which oil pulling plays a central role in both the prevention and the treatment of illness.

Ayurveda dates back to prehistoric times, to as early as 3000 BC. The word itself is a combination of *ayus,* "life," and *veda,* "knowledge." Thus the ayurvedic system is based on the "knowledge of life," a perspective that well agrees with the principles of traditional Indian medicine: that the medical arts and the art of living are one and the same. Because the concepts of ayurveda encompass all aspects of daily life, they can be applied equally on both healthy and sick days.

Ayurveda formed the basis of many healing systems outside of India, including traditional Chinese medicine (TCM). Our Western medicine has also been decisively influenced by ayurvedic insights, for it has been said that the treatment methods of the Hippocratic physicians were closely based on many of the principles of classical Indian medicine. Ayurveda's reputation as the "Mother of Medicine" is still acknowledged in our time. Although the traditional medicine of the Indian subcontinent was suppressed from 1858 to 1947 under the British Raj, ayurveda has reemerged today as an essential part of the Indian system of health care. And with our growing interest in all types of natural healing methods in the West, the Mother of Medicine has come to play an important role here as well. This has led to many scientific investigations of the efficacy of various ayurvedic therapies. The results of these investigations demonstrate that ayurveda has enormous potential as a modern system of holistic medicine that can be used to successfully treat a number of illnesses for which Western medicine has not yet found a cure.

❧

Dr. Fedor Karach

Many people who have searched the Internet to learn more about oil pulling have repeatedly encountered one name: Dr. Fedor Karach, a physician from the Ukraine. Dr. Karach claimed to have learned a simple and very effective health practice from Siberian shamans: each morning for at least four weeks in a row, one spoonful of sunflower oil should be thoroughly "chewed" and swished and sucked through the teeth and around the mouth for at least ten minutes, after which you spit the liquid out (being careful not to swallow any) and brush the teeth as usual. This practice could draw out and remove all kinds of harmful toxins, including even heavy metals, from the body. This corresponded to a similar ayurvedic technique, except that sesame oil is used in ayurveda, and the oil is swished for only about two minutes.

Dr. Karach gave a lecture about this practice of oil pulling during a late-1980s meeting of a group known as the "All-Ukrainian Association," which was attended by a number of oncologists and bacteriologists who were members of the Academy of Sciences of the USSR. The title of his presentation was "One of the Many Possibilities to Provide Assistance to an Ill or No Longer So Healthy Body." At the time, the practice of oil pulling was not well known in the West. The reaction to this presentation by those in attendance was overwhelmingly positive. Of course, there were also critics, but the main message did not go unheard.

It should be underscored that this time-tested health practice described by Dr. Karach to his colleagues did not originate in Russian or Ukrainian folk medicine, although oil pulling goes back centuries in the traditional medicine of those countries. All Dr. Karach did was remind those of us in the West about something that has been known and practiced in India and China for a long, long time.

The Five Elements and the Three Types

The basic assumption of ayurveda is that all of nature is composed of one or a combination of the five elements of ether, air, fire, water, and earth, and that all five of these elements are found within the human body. As well, from the perspective of traditional Indian medicine, everything that exists is in interrelationship with everything else. As a result, the diagnostic methods of ayurveda are complex and not based solely on the examination of a person's physical body; they also consider a number of other factors, such as the person's psychological state, lifestyle, and nutritional status, and even the climate in which the person lives.

The second principle of ayurveda is the doctrine of the three *doshas: vata, pitta,* and *kapha.* The Sanskrit term *dosha* can be translated as "support," a term that indicates its function; the doshas can be understood as the biological principles or bioenergies that support and control all of an organism's processes. Because the relationship between the doshas is established for each person at the time of birth, the ayurvedic system assumes that people have different constitutional types. These types make it possible to identify and address a person's health weaknesses and strengths.

The Five Treatments for Maintaining Health

All of the treatment methods used in ayurveda aim at maintaining or restoring the balance of the three doshas, the three supports. One of the methods involves the use of plant medicines—phytotherapy, in fact, plays a central role in the ayurvedic healing canon. Ayurvedic plant medicines are manufactured in a traditional manner and are based on recipes that have been passed down for centuries.

Ayurveda also makes use of purifying therapies intended to maintain or restore a person's health. The most important of these are the *panchakarma,* the "five treatments." These techniques, which are now recognized and practiced in the West, consist of a finely tuned system of purifying treatments and oil massages. One of these is *gandusha,* the ayurvedic practice of oil pulling.

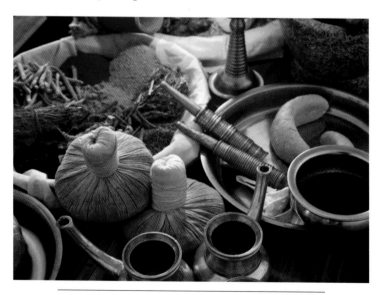

Herbs and oils play an important role in the various
treatments of ayurvedic medicine.

As the name itself suggests, the panchakarma are divided into five cycles, each of which is subdivided into a preparatory and a recovery phase. As the panchakarma are applied, the metabolic wastes and toxins in the tissues and organs are mobilized, enabling them to be more readily excreted or broken down by the body. This thorough "housecleaning" exerts enormously positive effects on all levels—physical, emotional, and mental. The intensive elimination and purification of harmful residues and waste products leads to an increase in the activity of the immune system and the restoration of balance in the nervous and endocrine systems. In addition, the panchakarma improve the circulation of the blood and strengthen the functioning of the organs. These are only some of the reasons why these treatments have long demonstrated themselves to be so useful in the prevention and treatment of so many illnesses. Later in this book we will more closely explore why therapies for purification and detoxification like panchakarma and oil pulling have such good results.

Gandusha—the Ayurvedic Practice of Oil Pulling

Ayurvedic oil pulling generally utilizes warm sesame oil or ghee (clarified butter). The ayurvedic method of oil pulling does not differ in any significant manner from oil pulling as we know it here in the West. However, traditional Indian medicine suggests that a person should first carry out certain preparatory steps. Before performing gandusha you should take some of the sesame oil or ghee to be used in the gandusha in your hands and softly rub it on your cheeks and neck. After that you saturate a small hand towel with warm water and with it remove the oil or ghee from the skin. This prepares the body for the gandusha so that its effects can more fully manifest.

The length of time that one should practice ayurvedic oil pulling differs from one person to the next. One sign that it has achieved its effects are tears in the eyes and a slight running of the nose; in some people this may occur sooner, while in others it may take more time.

Oil Swishing for Health

Oil swishing—another name for *oil pulling*—has long been practiced beyond the borders of India. One place where it has been practiced is Tibet, the "Roof of the World." As well, the people of the Middle Kingdom—the metaphorical name for China—have also known about and made use of this knowledge for many centuries. As in ayurvedic Indian medicine, traditional Chinese medicine (TCM) continues to make use of oil pulling to prevent and to treat illnesses.

This oil-based system of maintaining health also made its way into Russian folk medicine, especially in Belarus and the Ukraine, regions known for longevity, where it is and has long been held in high regard. Typical among the healing traditions of these regions is the use of simple treatment methods, especially among those who lived in the vast stretches of Russia. Few of these people lived near doctors or pharmacies, and among those who did, only the upper classes could actually afford such "luxuries." And so common people looked for other healing methods and remedies, and it was important that these be accessible and affordable to all. Both the Russian healers and those lay health practitioners who treated people found many of their treatments in nature—in the plant kingdom, in beekeeping, through agriculture, and in the earth. In addition, water and stones, and even the sun and the rain, were used as medicines. But most Russian folk remedies came from the kitchen. Knowing this, it is easy to understand how cooking oils came to be used for maintaining health. In the Russian folk medicine of our times, sunflower oil is still regarded as the best oil for oil pulling. But other oils are also suitable for this purpose, as we shall see later in this book.

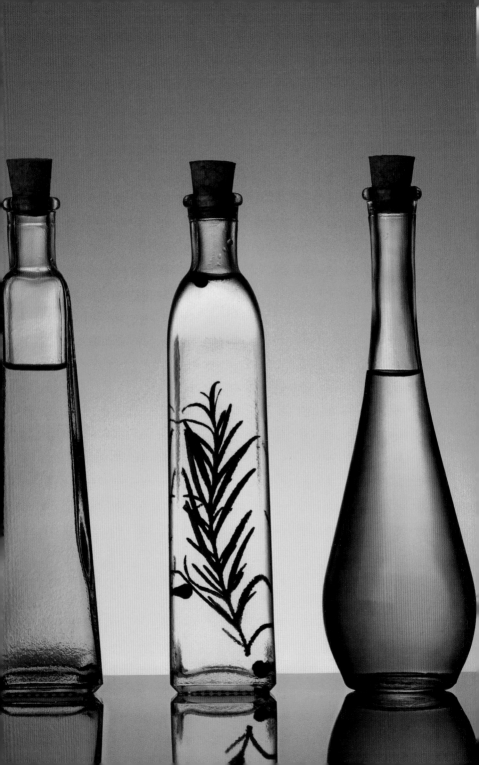

Oil Pulling for Body, Mind, and Spirit

There are many reasons behind oil pulling's long history of success. The health-promoting effects of pulling oil manifest throughout the body as well as mentally and emotionally. This is all the more remarkable when we consider how easy it is to pull oil!

The reasons why and how this simple method is able to produce such significant health benefits, as well as the specific effects it can have, will be discussed here. First, however, we should consider why detoxification and purification are so important for maintaining and restoring our health.

Regular Cleansing Boosts Our Health

Even if you have not been bitten by a poisonous snake or ingested arsenic, the body's detoxification system can still be frequently overwhelmed. An excess of unhealthy foods (including alcohol), stress, and especially the modern environmental toxins we are exposed to on a daily basis take their toll. A great number of illnesses can be attributed to the many years of collected toxins and waste products that accrue in the body. That's why it's important that the body be given a regular housecleaning.

The Body's Cleaning Crews

The liver is the body's primary detoxification station. This organ breaks down alcohol in the blood, as well as metabolic products, unmetabolized medications, and other harmful substances, and it neutralizes these pathogens and toxins. Everything that the body does not need or that could cause it harm is absorbed and neutralized by the liver and is expelled via the digestive and urinary tracts, the skin, and the breath. The kidneys too are a vital member of our full-time cleaning crew. They eliminate waste products through urine while conserving everything that we need for our bodies to function—everything that should not "go down the drain."

But the liver and kidneys are not only the organs that are responsible for keeping our internal affairs in order and thus keeping us healthy. Various metabolic processes play an important role. The complex machinery of the different metabolic processes—cellular respiration, fat metabolism, the Krebs cycle, glycolysis, and so forth—is responsible for the absorption and use of nutrients obtained through digestion. These processes also produce the energy that keeps us going. Additionally, and equally important, these metabolic processes are involved in the excretion of toxins and other harmful substances.

The lymphatic system is also an important member of the body's cleaning crew, for this finely branching network that

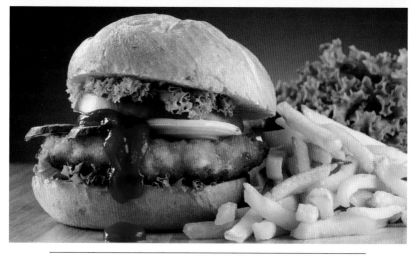

Fast food should be avoided as much as possible, as the combination of harmful fats and carbohydrates found in these foods can place a great burden on the body.

runs throughout the body is a transportation system that serves many functions. After the circulatory system, the lymphatic system is in fact our second most important means of transporting materials throughout the body. Lymphatic fluid, or lymph, helps to supply all of the body's cells with nutrients. But the lymphatic system plays an even greater role in cleansing, for the numerous branches of the lymphatic vascular system help remove metabolic end products, toxins, and other harmful substances, as well as other pathogens, from our bodies.

Unfortunately, the powers of our body's cleaning crew are not unlimited. This is the crux of the matter: everything that the liver, kidneys, and their colleagues cannot remove will remain in the body. And this can often have negative consequences.

The Body's Trash Dump

Our bodies have to do much more than simply digest the nutrients found in our daily meals. In these modern times they also have to handle the many food additives and preservatives found in food and the heavy metals and hormones that are present both in the environment and in many of our foods and personal products. In addition, many people consume nicotine, alcohol, and various kinds of drugs and pharmaceuticals. Moreover, we are exposed to vast amounts of acids, while an increasing number of environmental toxins assault us on a daily basis. This results in an accumulation of a variety of substances that can harm the body over time.

Our body's trash collectors have to dispose of all of these substances, and they do this twenty-four hours a day. But when they are overwhelmed with work they become unable to fulfill their duties adequately. This can cause bottlenecks in the metabolic and excretory processes. Our bodies solve such problems by stowing these substances away, preferably where they cannot cause any immediate harm: first in our connective tissues and fat cells, and then in our tendons, muscles, and joints. Remember that the most important task of our body's cleaning crew is to protect our vital organs from harm. In the pursuit of this goal, they are often forced to turn to less sensitive places to store toxic waste.

Eventually, however, even these deposits need to be neutralized. The body accomplishes this by mixing basic (as opposed to acidic) minerals and trace elements in the accumulated toxins. In this way the material that has collected in these secondary storage sites is transformed into metabolic wastes, which lie latent in the body. But latent does not necessarily mean harmless, for if these waste products are not removed on a regular basis the body can gradually change until it becomes in effect a trash dump. To prevent this, our intestines, skin, kidneys, liver, and even our breathing apparatus must work hard to detoxify and excrete these wastes. But if the liver, kidneys, intestines, skin, and breath have too much to do, they can reach their limits. These difficulties are compounded by the fact that our body's cleaning crews become less efficient as we age. As a result, the concentration of waste products in the body tends to increase over time. A variety of health issues can arise as the body becomes overburdened with these metabolic wastes and toxins; these complaints include food allergies, chronic fatigue, a weakened immune system, digestive problems, a decline in mental performance, and much more.

The Adverse Effects of Old Waste Deposits

As environmentalists often point out, trash dumps are fraught with dangers. It is no different in our bodies. Here, too, the waste sites in our connective tissues, fat cells, and joints can pose an enormous risk.

Let's begin by considering the intestines, which are often regarded as the seat of health. Many of the body's waste products and toxins may become trapped in the intestines' multitude of undulations and convolutions, creating an especially high burden on this organ. This can hinder the abilities of the intestinal villi, whose job it is to absorb nutrients from the chime, the semifluid mass of food, enzymes, and other materials that travel from the stomach to the large intestine. Over time this can lead to lapses in the absorption of vitamins, minerals, and trace elements. In addition, these old waste products can create a fatal breeding ground for germs and fungi. At first these can grow without creating any noticeable symptoms, but over time they can undermine the very basis of our health and vitality.

The Root of Health

The Austrian physician Franz Xaver Mayr (1875–1965) referred to the intestines as "the root of health." Mayr is primarily known for developing the Franz Xaver Mayr Cure, also known as Mayr Therapy. The important role that healthy intestines and therefore good digestion play in our well-being has been known since antiquity. The physicians of ancient Greece determined that "all evils dwell in the intestine."

The substances that can cause illness have ample room to dwell in our intestines. This organ measures an impressive 22.9 feet (7 meters) in length. If we could flatten out the innumerable evaginations and villi of its mucous membranes, the resulting area would cover approximately half of a football field. These dimensions reflect the importance of the processes that occur within the intestinal tract, processes that are not only responsible for our feelings of satiety but also serve to maintain our overall health. The intestines also play an important role as part of the immune system, as the mucous membranes that line the entire digestive tract contribute to protect us against diseases.

The immune system can also suffer from an excess of bodily wastes. The lymphatic system, which as we have already seen plays an important role in waste disposal, may not be able to keep up with the demands that are being placed on it. Because this system of transportation is a crucial component of our line of defense, the effectiveness of the immune system may be significantly impaired. The resulting negative impacts may be as threatening as when the intestines become overburdened with metabolic wastes.

The damage that occurs when large amounts of waste products are lodged in the muscles and joints results in arthritis and refractory muscle tension. These conditions are not simply the result of wear and tear or excessive use alone—excessive waste deposits lodged there are frequently the culprit behind painful joints and tense muscles.

Last but not least, waste products that are deposited in the body's connective tissues also lead to problems. Cellulite, that dreaded and well-known condition that seems to affect women in particular, is just one of the end results that occur when the connective tissues are mired in waste products. The

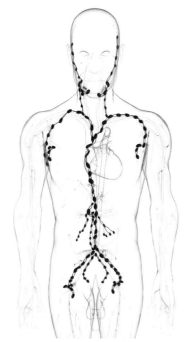

The lymphatic system

body's ability to transmit information from nerve cell to nerve cell can also be impaired.

Clearly, we should do everything we can to remove these harmful and illness-causing wastes from our bodies. And one of the most effective ways to do this is by oil pulling.

Healthy on All Levels

Oil pulling has many beneficial effects on our physical, mental, and emotional health. What is behind these positive effects? As a result of the growing interest in ancient healing modalities like ayurveda, in recent years a number of scientific studies have been conducted on the efficacy of oil pulling in maintaining health and healing various illnesses.* What we can glean from the results of these studies is that just as the effects of many natural remedies, especially medicinal plants, can be attributed to a number of different factors, the wide-ranging beneficial effects of oil pulling are also due to a variety of mechanisms. Let us now take a closer look at these

---

*An overview of the kinds of studies that have been conducted in recent years on the efficacy of oil pulling includes the following: F. C. Peedikayil, P. Sreenivasan, and A. Narayanan, "Effect of coconut oil in plaque related gingivitis—a preliminary report," *Nigerian Medical Journal* 56, no. 2 (2015): doi:10.4103/0300-1652; P. Sood, M. A. Devi, R. Narang, et al., "Comparative efficacy of oil pulling and chlorhexidine on oral malodor: A randomized controlled trial," *Journal of Clinical and Diagnostic Research* 8, no. 11 (2014): 18–21; A. Singh and B. Purohit, "Tooth brushing, oil pulling and tissue regeneration: A review of holistic approaches to oral health," *Journal of Ayurveda and Integrative Medicine* 2, no. 2 (2011): 64–68; and S. Asokan, T. K. Rathinasamy, N. Inbamani, et al., "Mechanism of oil-pulling therapy—in vitro study," *Indian Journal of Dental Research* 22, no. 1 (2011): 34–37.

"multifactorial mechanisms of action," as they are known in science.

The Oral Mucosae

Oil pulling, as we know, occurs in the mouth, so first we need to know that the mucous membranes in the mouth play an important role in the purging of waste from the body. The basic function of the oral mucosae is to moisten food with secretions from the glands. These secretions contain enzymes that are responsible for the first stage of digestion. However, the oral mucosae also do something else that is of vital importance: they secrete metabolic wastes as well as harmful and toxic substances.

The important role that the oral mucosae play in detoxification and purification can also be seen when we fast. Abstaining from food causes toxins and wastes to be liberated from the tissues and fat cells. Once freed, these substances collect on the tongue, where they can be seen as deposits that are often quite thick and slimy. Scraping the tongue or otherwise removing these deposits is an important activity that contributes to maintaining health, and this technique is discussed in more detail later in this book. Because the tongue is also covered in mucous membranes, the coating that appears on it provides a clear indication of the role that the oral mucosae play in our body's waste removal process.

The coating on your tongue will vary considerably depending on the state of your health. Practitioners of traditional healing systems such as ayurveda and traditional Chinese medicine (TCM) look carefully at the tongue when diagnosing health problems. For example, in TCM a swollen tongue with a white greasy coating indicates water retention in the body, while a cracked red tongue with little or no coating indicates a deficiency of yin energy, as is commonly seen during menopause.

How Oil Pulls Harmful Substances from the Body

Oil pulling involves pulling a small amount of oil back and forth between the teeth and throughout the entire oral cavity for a period of time that can range from a few minutes to twenty minutes or so. As this action is performed, the oil literally pulls plaque, toxins, and metabolic waste products out of the body. How is this accomplished? Oil possesses the ability to bind with other substances, and not only those that may be harmful. Although fat-soluble substances are especially amenable to this process, oils can also remove water-soluble substances. The back-and-forth swishing of oil in the mouth creates an emulsion, an oil-water mixture in which tiny droplets of water are suspended. In this way, oil pulling helps to remove both water-soluble and fat-soluble wastes from our bodies.

In other words, everything that our glands secrete through our oral mucosae can be absorbed and eliminated by the oil. Because our excretory functions operate at full speed during the night, a high concentration of our body's wastes accumulate in the oral cavity while we are sleeping. This is why the best time to practice oil pulling is in the morning, upon arising.

But the oil that you pull through your mouth does more than just remove the substances that are present in your oral mucosae. The intense movement of the oil in the mouth powerfully stimulates the flow of blood to the glands located in the oral cavity, and this in turn leads to a substantial increase in their activity. In this way, even more harmful substances are eliminated from the body as the glands, stimulated by an increased flow of blood, begin to flush. In other words, oil pulling initiates a type of deep cleaning action by which even more deep-seated toxins and harmful materials may be drawn into the mouth and then excreted. The result is a marked increase in the cleansing effects.

As this is occurring, the salivary glands that serve the oral mucosae are also stimulated, further strengthening the immune system. Saliva contains proteins that are essential for protecting us against pathogens. These include immunoglobulin A, which binds to all kinds of disease-causing germs, and lysozymes that dissolve bacterial cell walls, thereby rendering them harmless. The more of these and other such protective agents that are present in the saliva, the better equipped we are to resist the onslaught of pathogens.

The intensive rinsing of the mouth with oil has remarkable effects that can be felt throughout the entire body. When the glands in the oral mucosae are stimulated, enzymes are released that directly activate the functions of various organs and tissues in the body. One effect of this is an intensification of the entire body's efforts to rid itself of toxins. Thus oil pulling triggers the mouth to signal other parts of the body that they should start getting rid of their accumulated wastes. This brings us to another aspect of how pulling keeps us healthy, and this touches on the close relationship between the teeth and the various regions and organs of the body.

What the Microscope Brings to Light

We can see how effectively oil pulling works to remove all manner of harmful and unnecessary substances by looking at saliva through a microscope. A close-up examination reveals substantial amounts of toxins, bacteria, and other pathogens in the average person's saliva. For example, scientific studies have confirmed that oil pulling effectively protects against *Streptococcus mutans*.* When the oil used for pulling was examined under a microscope, it was found to contain large numbers of these bacteria, which have been found to be one of the most significant contributors to dental cavities.

---

*S. Asokan, J. Rathan, M. S. Muthu, et al., "Effect of oil pulling on *Streptococcus mutans* count in plaque and saliva using Dentocult SM Strip mutans test: A randomized, controlled, triple-blind study," *Journal of the Indian Society of Pedodontics and Preventative Dentistry* 26, no. 1 (2008): 12–17.

The Connection between the Body and the Teeth

Integrated, or holistic, dentistry recognizes that our teeth are directly connected to certain organs and body parts in a kind of microcosmic-macrocosmic relationship. It employs this knowledge by using the teeth and their condition to therapeutically treat the different body parts and organs with which they are associated.

The notion that there is a connection between the nerves and blood vessels in the teeth and the rest of the body is not far-fetched. The thin root canal that serves each individual

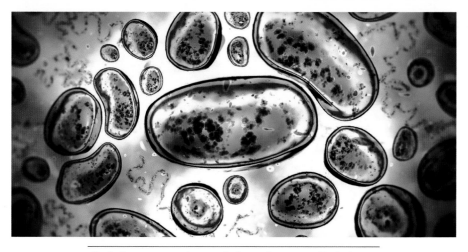

Bacteria as seen under an electron microscope. Bacteria are living organisms that occur in very different forms.

tooth contains nerves and blood vessels that originate in the jaw and, in turn, are extensions of the same web of nerves and blood vessels that connect to other parts of the body. Our understanding of this holistic relationship between the body and the mouth comes from traditional Chinese medicine. TCM moreover considers the role that both individual teeth as well as the entire oral cavity have in regulating our body's functions. TCM assigns our organs and all our other body parts to different bodily functions that are energetically interconnected with one another. Such healing treatments as acupuncture and acupressure, as well as the ancient healing practice of qigong, can be used to target a specific functional entity so as to restore and preserve its health. Of all the functional entities recognized by TCM, only two do not have any correspondences in the mouth.

Just as TCM divides the feet into different reflex zones that correspond to different parts of the body and different functions, and uses different massage or acupuncture techniques to influence them, TCM similarly divides the

Body-Mouth Correspondences

- Bladder: upper and lower first and second incisors
- Large intestine (colon): upper first and second premolars; lower first and second molars
- Small intestine: upper and lower third molars ("wisdom teeth")
- Gallbladder: upper and lower canines as well as the sides of the tongue
- Heart: upper and lower molars as well as the tongue, especially the tip
- Liver: upper and lower canines as well as both sides of the tongue
- Lungs: upper first and second premolars; lower first and second molars; tip of the tongue and the throat region
- Stomach: upper first and second molars; lower first and second premolars; middle of the tongue and the gums
- Spleen: upper left first and second molars; bottom left first and second premolars; middle of the tongue
- Kidneys: upper and lower first and second incisors as well as the root of the tongue

tongue into different reflex zones that correspond to different parts of the body and their functions. As a result of this holistic connection between the teeth and the rest of the body, it is assumed that the intensive back-and-forth swishing of oil in the mouth elicits stimuli that can exert an influence on the corresponding body areas and organs. Again, this is the

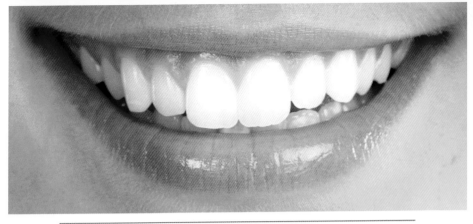

The integrated approach of traditional Chinese medicine assigns different teeth to specific organs, pains, and associated emotions.

same principle that underlies the practices of acupuncture and acupressure, in which specific points on the meridians are stimulated in order to exert therapeutic effects on distant but related parts of the body.

Defusing the "Time Bombs" in Our Mouths

The potential problems that can develop in our mouths over time, which may correspond to problems in related organs of the body, as noted above, may remain undetected for a long period of time, just as toxins accumulate over time. Although they may be not clearly visible, what are known as *dental foci*—oral sources of infection that affect other areas and organs in the body—can lead to massive disturbances in our health.

Dental foci are pockets of pathogens and inflammation found deep within the bones of the jaw. They form near the roots of the teeth, which reach deep into the bony regions and the lacunae (small cavities, pits, or discontinuities in the anatomical structure) of the jaws. The circulation of blood in these areas is poor, which means that the body's defense systems only rarely patrol these regions. This creates an ideal condition for harmful germs and bacteria to establish themselves and exert their destructive effects. These foci may also contain toxins, harmful metabolic products, and residues of medicines, all of which can lead to pockets of inflammation in the teeth. Such oral time bombs can also develop following a tooth extraction if remnants of the tooth are inadvertently left in the jawbone.

If unrecognized by a dentist, dental foci can cause damage to nearby teeth, and the toxins and harmful pathogens they constantly exude can create problems for the body's metabolic processes and challenge the immune system. What's more, these dental foci can affect the circulatory and nervous systems and the lymphatic fluid, leading to serious problems in other organs and tissues, even those far removed from the mouth. The afflicted areas can cause chronic inflammation and irritation throughout the body, and the consequences of this continuous strain on our health can be severe. It is not surprising that holistic dental care and naturopathic medicine place a great deal of emphasis on eradicating dental foci.

When dental foci are present, oil pulling can provide a great deal of help. Because oil aids in transporting harmful microbial secretions out of the entire mouth and pharynx, and secondarily affects corresponding organs of the body, the technique of oil pulling can help defuse these oral time bombs and thereby significantly decrease their potentially dangerous effects. Oil, when swished through the mouth, helps remove the very substances that these pockets of pathogens would otherwise release into the body. In this way, oil pulling gets to the root of this problem—in this case, the roots of the teeth.

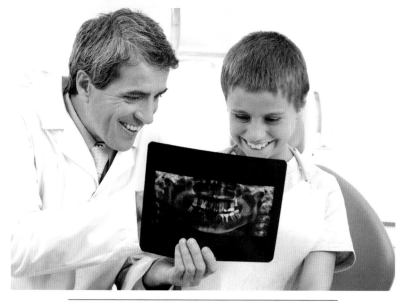

X-rays play an important role in recognizing and treating illnesses that can affect our teeth.

An Essential Component of Holistic Healing

For the same reasons that it can be so useful in treating dental foci and resulting health problems, oil pulling is one of the most effective and time-honored methods for staying healthy, preventing illness, and maintaining well-being. Simply put, oil pulling supports our body's innate ability to heal itself and to stay healthy. Dr. Fedor Karach made note of this in his groundbreaking 1980s talk, in which he introduced the practice of oil pulling to Russian scientists: "The actual healing is initiated by the body," he explained. "In this way, it is possible to heal cells, tissues, and all organs simultaneously."

The astonishing thing about oil pulling is that its effects are more than just preventive, although it is very much a preventive health technique. Even when a person's body has been overburdened with harmful toxins and waste products, and illnesses are manifesting as a result, oil pulling can help. The ability of oil pulling to mobilize our innate self-healing powers can be seen in both acute ailments and chronic illnesses. In other words, whether you want to treat a health problem that has just arisen or an illness that has been affecting you for some time, oil pulling is something that you might want to consider. And if you want to avoid illnesses and support your health and well-being, oil pulling can be a valuable adjunct to your wellness regimen.

Oil Pulling Is Not a Panacea

The list of ailments that oil pulling has helped to alleviate is considerable. You will get a better idea as to the scope of the conditions that will benefit from this method when you look at the list below. Nevertheless, this naturopathic treatment method is not a panacea, nor should it be considered as one.

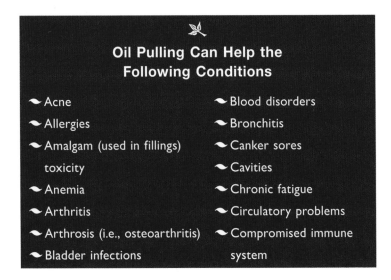

Oil Pulling Can Help the Following Conditions

- Acne
- Allergies
- Amalgam (used in fillings) toxicity
- Anemia
- Arthritis
- Arthrosis (i.e., osteoarthritis)
- Bladder infections
- Blood disorders
- Bronchitis
- Canker sores
- Cavities
- Chronic fatigue
- Circulatory problems
- Compromised immune system

- Conjunctivitis
- Constipation
- Coughing
- Debilitation (weakness, lassitude)
- Depression
- Difficulties concentrating
- Digestive difficulties
- Ear pain
- Ear-nose-throat ailments
- Eczema
- Eye disorders
- Failing eyesight
- Fatigue
- Flatulence
- Flu infections
- Gastritis
- Gingivitis
- Gynecological illnesses
- Headaches
- Heart problems
- Herpes
- Hoarseness
- Infections
- Intestinal disorders
- Jaw and sinus infections and secretions
- Kidney ailments
- Liver disease
- Loose teeth
- Loss of appetite
- Lung disease
- Menopausal complaints
- Menstrual complaints
- Migraines
- Mucosal ailments
- Nerve ailments
- Nervous conditions
- Neurodermatitis (itchy-skin condition usually found in nervous people)
- Overstimulation
- Paralytic symptoms
- Periodontal problems
- Premenstrual syndrome
- Psoriasis
- Rheumatic complaints
- Skin impurities
- Sleep disturbances
- Sniffling
- Sore throat
- Stomach ulcers
- Thrombosis
- Tonsillitis
- Tooth discoloration
- Toothache
- Urinary incontinence
- Withdrawal symptoms, especially from nicotine

It is true that oil pulling can be used to effectively treat a number of ailments. What is more, based on his observations of Siberian shamans, Dr. Karach reasoned that oil pulling could actually extend a person's life span, and he argued that it is entirely possible for humans to live for well over a hundred years. Though we have no way of knowing definitively whether regular oil pulling can account for such longevity as what Dr. Karach observed in the Siberian practitioners of this method, what we do know is that oil pulling has helped many people deal with a wide variety of health issues. We know that oil pulling has been practiced since ancient times, by various cultures, and for good reason. But this does not make it a substitute for a visit to your doctor or health care practitioner. Avoiding medical attention is not and cannot be the goal of this ancient healing modality.

Why Oil Pulling Works

Oil pulling is able to exert such comprehensive beneficial effects on our health because it:

- Provides an intensive and long-lasting detoxification and purification of the body
- Strengthens the body's own defenses
- Stimulates the body's self-healing powers in a powerful way
- Leads to lasting improvements in our physical, mental, and emotional states

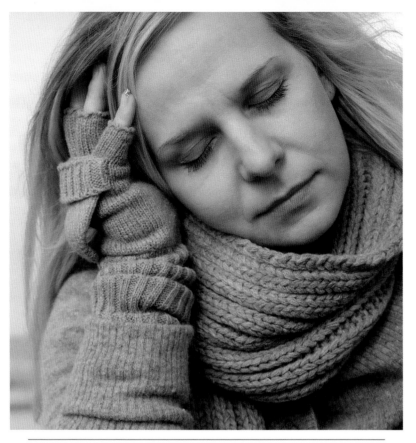

Oil pulling can also help prevent the flu.

Should I Pull Oil?

Recently, I have been tired a lot and unable to bring myself to do things. I also get headaches more frequently. And I have not been sleeping very well lately. Maybe this is why I have been in such a bad mood and overly irritable . . .

Does this sound familiar? Or have you noticed other things occurring that amount to you just not feeling very well? In most cases, pulling oil can help.

A Health Issues Checklist

To determine whether you might want to try pulling oil, see if you can answer many of the following questions in this checklist in the affirmative:

- Are you frequently constipated?
- Do you tend to have flatulence?
- Do you have problems sleeping through the night?
- Are you more prone to infections lately?
- Are your breathing passages often inflamed?
- Do you frequently have dark thoughts or suffer from depression?
- Do you get oral herpes frequently?
- Do your gums bleed?
- Are you irritable?
- Do you have stomach problems?
- Do you have skin problems?
- Do you have frequent headaches?
- Do you suffer from joint pain?
- Do you often find it difficult to concentrate?
- Do you get cramps in your calves?
- Do you have tight muscles, especially in the neck?
- Do you quickly develop dental tartar?
- Do you catch colds easily?
- Do you often feel tired and worn out?
- Do stressful situations affect you more severely than they used to?
- Do you have problems digesting foods that you were previously able to digest?

➤ Do you suffer from neurodermatitis (itchy skin) or psoriasis?

➤ Has your vision deteriorated for no apparent reason?

➤ Do you often suffer from a loss of appetite?

➤ Are you nervous and tense?

➤ Do you have heart problems?

➤ Do you suffer from frequent bladder infections?

➤ Do you wish to stop smoking?

➤ Are your teeth discolored?

➤ Are your teeth loose?

If you experience any or many of these conditions, oil pulling may help.

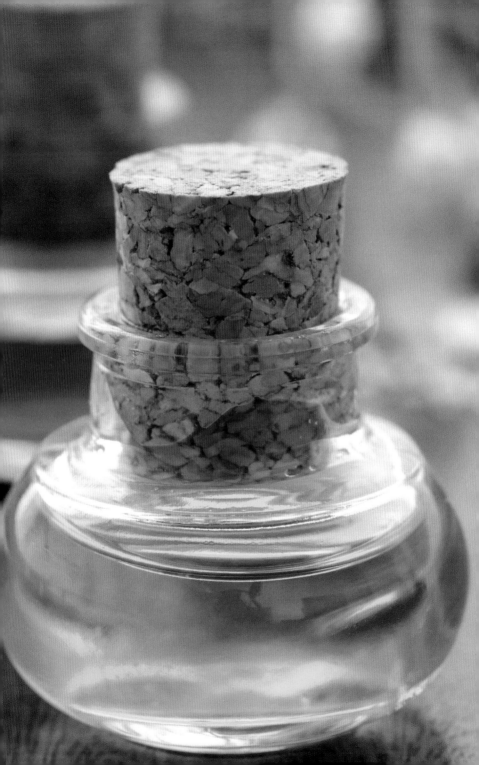

Five Minutes a Day
for Your Well-Being

Oil pulling is really a very simple process. You can do it at any time, without any special knowledge or preparation. All that is needed is five minutes of your time. And as you will see, this is time well invested.

Once Daily—Your Cure

Despite the simplicity of the technique, you should still understand the steps involved in oil pulling. Otherwise, you may make some small mistakes that could reduce the success of your efforts.

When Should I Pull Oil?

In principle, you can pull oil at any time of the day, but the best time is in the morning, just after waking up. This is because during the night, waste products, toxins, and other harmful substances accumulate in the oral mucosae. In the morning, these can be removed en masse with just one swish of oil.

Before pulling oil, avoid drinking coffee, juice, or even water. Otherwise, you could wash a good portion of what you want to expel back into your body, as first thing in the morning the toxins are ready and waiting to be expelled. Therefore, you should pull oil before putting anything in your mouth. If you wish, you may want to turn on your coffeemaker or tea kettle before you begin. This way, you can look forward to the first cup of the day while you are pulling and swishing. In some cases, such as when you are dealing with a persistent chronic illness and wish to accelerate the healing process, you can pull oil three times day, including first thing in the morning. If you do, just as you would when swishing in the morning, it is important that you pull oil *before* eating.

To Begin

Put a spoonful of oil in your mouth. One full tablespoon is best. If this is too much, then use only one teaspoon, but no less. Starting with this amount, you can gradually work your way up to a full tablespoon. This amount is preferable because it allows the oil pulling to accomplish its full effects, which in part have to do with the physical and mechanical stimulation made possible by a certain quantity of oil. Children as young as six can pull oil. One teaspoon is enough for small children. Older children can work up to the adult dose.

Pull and Swish Vigorously

After taking the oil into your mouth, be sure to keep it in constant motion: suck it through your teeth, chew it, and swish it around your mouth. Relax while you are doing this and avoid tensing up or cramping the muscles of your mouth;

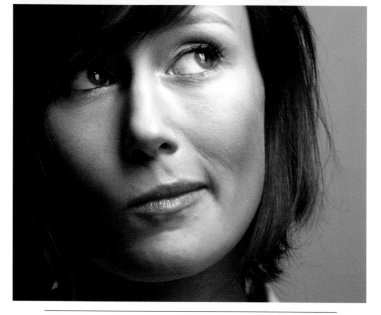

The oil should be slowly swished around in the mouth and sucked through the teeth for five minutes.

otherwise many of the healing effects of oil pulling can be lost. In other words, it's the difference between sipping tea and gulping it—you want to be steady and relaxed as you swish the oil around in your mouth.

Don't be surprised when the consistency of the oil changes in your mouth while you are oil pulling. As it combines with your saliva, the oil will become progressively less viscous. The

If You Wear Dentures

You can still pull oil effectively if you wear full or partial dentures; however, be sure to remove them before you begin to pull oil. Because dentures cover a large part of the oral mucosae, leaving them in would prevent the oil from reaching many of the areas that it should and thereby reduce the effectiveness of this therapy.

foamy mixture that develops is completely normal and even desirable.

Do Not Swallow

While you are pulling oil, you should hold your head straight or, better yet, tilted slightly forward. In any case, avoid leaning your head back as if you were gargling, for doing so increases the chances of swallowing some of the liquid. This should be strictly avoided; after all, the idea is to *expel* the harmful substances that have bound themselves to the oil and not *ingest* them. But if you do accidentally swallow some of the liquid, don't worry. It won't harm you; it just means that you have not completely purged yourself of these substances. In such a case the toxins and wastes that you accidentally swallowed will enter your digestive system and make their way back into your blood via the small intestine. These can then be disposed of the next time you pull oil.

Out with the Bad

Oil pulling should be performed for about five minutes.* When you spit out the oil, it should be milky white or at least pale yellow. If it is still greenish yellow, then you did not swish for long enough. After spitting out the oil, rinse out your mouth several times with warm water. Finally, brush with a toothbrush as you would normally.

It is sometimes advised that the oil should be spat into the toilet bowl, as this is where we typically dispose of our

---

*Some sources suggest pulling for longer periods, which is fine if you wish to do so, but in my opinion five minutes a day is quite sufficient.

bodily waste. However, it's fine to just spit the swished oil into the sink—just make sure that afterward you briefly wash out the sink, as the discarded fluid contains a multitude of toxins.

How Long before I See Results?

There are different opinions as to how long one must continue a daily regimen of oil pulling before seeing results. Of course, as we know, oil pulling can be done on a daily basis as a part of your regular stay-healthy routine, and in this case, if you are otherwise healthy, the benefits of oil pulling will be ongoing and perhaps not dramatic. On the other hand, many people with chronic or long-term illness who are using this technique to heal might wonder how long they will need to pull oil before experiencing its beneficial results. Dr. Karach was of the opinion that many acute complaints would begin to disappear after just two to four days of oil pulling. But in my opinion this is not realistic. My own experiences with oil pulling have shown me that more time—at least one week in the case of a short-term illness—is needed to truly achieve any noticeable effects. Obviously, if you have suffered from a chronic illness over a longer period of time, it will take longer to achieve noticeable results, and therefore the process will require more perseverance. Keep in mind that anything that has undermined and impaired your health over a period of time cannot be cured from one day to the next—even oil pulling cannot accomplish this. Therefore, when treating chronic, long-term illness with oil pulling, it is perfectly realistic to practice this method for a year or more before relief or healing of the condition occurs.

For those who are suffering from an illness, whether short- or long-term, the following signs will indicate that oil pulling is beginning to exert its positive effects:

- You are able to sleep well at night.
- You wake up in the morning refreshed and rested, without any bags under your eyes.
- You have a healthy appetite.

Generally, when you are suffering from an illness, it can take anywhere from four to six weeks until the full effects of oil pulling can be seen and the practice will have been able to exert a positive effect on all levels, physically, emotionally, and mentally. Consequently, it is recommended that you carry out a regimen of oil pulling for approximately six weeks during both the spring and the fall. However, this does not mean that oil pulling cannot be done daily, and indeed, this is the key to maintaining good health according to many people who have pulled oil for years.

Your Tongue and Your Health

Many ancient medical traditions such as ayurveda regard the tongue as an indicator of overall well-being. Based on the appearance of the tongue—whether swollen or wrinkled, uncoated or coated, and if coated, what the coating looks like—an ayurvedic practitioner can ascertain the cause of an illness. If the tongue is coated with a great deal of waste products consisting of dead cells, food remnants, and bacteria, the practitioner can make a conclusion about which organs are affected, for example, the stomach or digestive tract. Oftentimes a coating on the tongue can form because the person is not chewing

Massaging and Scraping

You may wish to augment your oil pulling routine with either or both of two other tried-and-true methods for cleansing the mouth and thereby your entire body. The first practice is gum massage; the second is tongue scraping. Both of these practices are performed after you brush your teeth.

To massage your gums, rub your fingers on the gums of your upper and lower jaws by moving them from the edges of your teeth toward the gums. Repeat this on all four sides of the mouth. Your fingers should apply only enough pressure to move your gums slightly without hurting them. This massage promotes the detoxification process and also stimulates circulation in the gums. This strengthens your gums and improves their abilities to resist harmful outside factors.

As already noted, the accumulation of waste matter and toxins in the body can lead to a coating on your tongue. This occurs with a variety of chronic illnesses, especially stomach and intestinal ailments. This biofilm should be removed on a regular basis. This can be done with a tea-

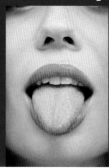

spoon, which you can use to scrape your tongue, working from the back of the tongue toward the tip. Rinse the scraped coating off the spoon and repeat the process two or three times. By now, the coating on your tongue should be gone.

Instead of a spoon, you can also use a special tongue scraper designed specifically for this purpose. These are also commonly used in ayurveda. Although such scrapers are typically made of wood, you may also choose one made out of stainless steel.

food well. On the other hand, a tongue with a cracked surface may indicate that the person has liver or stomach problems.

The reason why the tongue reveals so much about a person's health is at least in part due to the great role it plays in helping the body remove waste products and harmful substances. These wastes accumulate as layers on the tongue that can easily be removed. For this reason, cleaning the tongue of these waste products is an excellent adjunct to your regular morning regimen of oral care. (See the box "Massaging and Scraping").

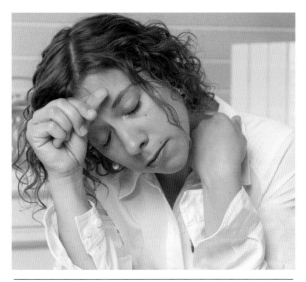

The beginning of an oil pulling cure can sometimes lead to a worsening of your symptoms—a good sign that the cure is working, as toxins are being released.

Possible Side Effects

As the detoxification process begins and your body is finally able to start ridding itself of old, harmful contaminants, you may exhibit any of the following temporary side effects:

- Fever
- Joint problems or stiffness
- Sore throat
- Swollen lymph nodes
- Mild flu-like symptoms
- Digestive problems, including constipation or diarrhea
- Headache, especially when the liver is detoxifying

You Might Feel Worse at First

Sometimes, what is known in holistic medicine as a *healing crisis* can occur soon after you begin pulling oil. This is a sign of detoxification that shows up as a worsening of your symptoms; in other words, the symptoms of an existing illness may become more pronounced or you may start to experience flu-like symptoms or a headache. It should be noted that such an initial phase of seemingly getting worse can also occur when you are using a homeopathic or other natural healing remedy, and it is actually seen as a positive sign. The initial—and temporary—deterioration is an indication that the process of the release of toxins from the body has begun. As this occurs, more deeply seated pockets of waste products and previously unrecognized foci of disease-causing substances are able to come to the surface. As the saying goes, "You cannot make an omelet without breaking some eggs." In the case of oil pulling, a healing crisis is a good sign that the process is working, and this initial reaction to the release of toxins should be no cause for alarm, nor should it cause you to stop pulling oil. To the contrary, these early symptoms are an indication that your steps toward better health are taking you in the right direction. Of course, if your worsening symptoms persist, seek the advice of your health care practitioner.

The Various Kinds of Oils

A number of different vegetable oils can be used for oil pulling. No matter which one you decide to use, you should always be sure to use only high-quality, cold-pressed vegetable oils. While these are admittedly more expensive than oils obtained through a different process, your health is well worth the price.

On the following pages you will find a selection from the rich assortment of health-promoting oils that can be used for oil pulling. In addition to their abilities to detoxify and purify the body, many of these oils also elicit more specific effects. The recommended oils to be used for oil pulling are described in alphabetical order.

Health by the Spoonful

Plant oils, which have a very good composition of fatty acids, literally serve up health by the spoonful. The building blocks of these oils are long chains of carbon atoms that can occur in three different forms: saturated, monounsaturated, and polyunsaturated fatty acids. Each of these affects our health in different ways. It is best to avoid saturated fatty acids, which are found primarily in animal fats. These fats carry an enormous risk, for they can elevate the level of LDL "bad" cholesterol in

A Short Primer on Oil

There are many types of oils, and they may be classified in different ways. Most of the terms below have to do with the ways in which the oils have been processed and their constituent components. It is important that you understand the meanings of these terms so that you can more carefully consider the oil that you will use for oil pulling.

❧ **Virgin** edible (or cooking) fats and oils are obtained from raw materials by milling or pressing these materials at a low temperature or through some other gentle mechanical process. After pressing, the material can be washed, filtered, or centrifuged; other procedures are not allowed. Olive oil and cocoa butter are subject to additional specific regulations.

❧ **Unrefined** edible fats and oils are obtained by rendering or through such gentle mechanical means as pressing and centrifugation. In contrast to virgin oils, unrefined oils may also be treated with water vapor and dried. However, these oils may not be deacidified, bleached, or deodorized.

❧ Virgin or unrefined edible oils that are labeled *cold-pressed* or *first cold-pressed* are considered to be the best. These are obtained through pressing without adding heat and by using the gentlest possible mechanical processes.

❧ The terms *edible oil*, *plant oil*, *table oil*, *salad oil*, and *frying oil* are all used to refer to mixtures of different oils in which the specific ingredients need not be listed. Many of the least expensive of these oils consist of mostly rapeseed oil or soy oil, while some of the more expensive name brands consist primarily of sunflower oil.

➤ If an oil bears the name of a specific plant, such as **sunflower oil,** at least 97 percent of that oil must come from that raw source.

➤ If such an oil is labeled **pure** or **unmixed,** then 100 percent of that oil must have been obtained from that raw source.

the blood, increasing the chances of cardiovascular illnesses. They can also disrupt fat metabolism.

What we do need are the good fats, those containing high amounts of unsaturated fatty acids. Monounsaturated fatty acids such as oleic acid lower the levels of LDL cholesterol, protect the heart and blood vessels, and help balance the metabolism. In contrast to monounsaturated fatty acids, polyunsaturated fatty acids can be broken along more points in their carbon chains. Among the polyunsaturated fatty acids are linoleic acid, linolenic acid, and alpha-linolenic acid. These correct the levels of fats in the blood by lowering the levels of harmful LDL cholesterol and increasing the levels of HDL "good" cholesterol. They also help lower blood pressure, provide protection against free radicals, and help reduce inflammation.

For these reasons, nutritionists recommend that we primarily use monounsaturated and polyunsaturated fatty acids to meet our dietary fat requirements—in other words, that we ingest sufficient quantities of plant oils.

Use Only Cold-Pressed Oils

Why is it important that the oil you use for pulling be cold-pressed? It is because these oils are only processed at low temperatures, hence the name. In this way the valuable constituents in the plant oils are preserved. In contrast, the processes that yield refined oils involve much higher temperatures, while extracting oils entails the use of chemical solvents.

What Are Cold-Pressed Oils?

The best oils are cold-pressed. Many types of fruits, seeds, and vegetables can be used to make cold-pressed oil, but not all cooking oils go through this process. The introduction of heat to the process of making commercial oils degrades their flavor, nutritional value, and color and may expose them to toxins.

For an oil to be considered cold-pressed, the oil is first obtained through pressing and grinding fruit or seeds with the use of heavy granite millstones or modern stainless steel presses, which are found in large commercial operations. Although pressing and grinding produces heat through friction, the temperature must not rise above 120°F (49°C) for any oil to be considered cold-pressed, and many cold-pressed oils are produced at even lower temperatures. Cold-pressed oils retain all of their flavor, aroma, and nutritional value.

Because of how they are produced, both refined and extracted oils have lost many of their beneficial effects. For this reason, such oils should not be used for oil pulling.

Canola Oil

The oil obtained from the seeds of the yellow-blooming rapeseed (*Brassica napus* subspecies *napus*) has only recently become available for culinary purposes. Although rapeseed (or rape) has been cultivated for its oil-bearing seeds for centuries, the erucic acid contained in wild rapeseed, as well as other extremely bitter substances, made the oil unpalatable. It was only during the 1980s that varieties of rapeseed containing only small amounts of erucic acid and bitters were successfully derived. This particular variety of rapeseed, which produces what is commonly called *canola oil* (or double-low rapeseed oil), has a favorable composition of fatty acids. To obtain the oil, the rapeseeds are cleaned, dried, and then pressed in oil mills at temperatures that may not exceed 104°F (40°C). Organic (only organic should be used to avoid contamination by GMOs) cold-pressed canola oil has a very pleasant spicy and nutty taste.

Storage and Shelf Life

Since it is very light-sensitive, canola oil must be stored in a cool, dark place. Open bottles are best stored sealed in the refrigerator. Once opened, the oil is best used within four to six weeks. In its original sealed container, canola oil can be stored for up to twelve months.

Effects

The composition of canola oil is optimal, with some 63 percent monounsaturated oleic acid, 36 percent polyunsaturated alpha-linolenic acid, and only 6 to 8 percent saturated fatty acids. It also contains vitamins A and E. Canola oil regulates fat metabolism and protects against such cardiovascular ill-nesses as atherosclerosis and heart attack.

Coconut Oil

The nuts—i.e., the fruit—of the coconut palm (*Cocos nucifera*) yield an oil that is becoming increasingly popular for maintaining and restoring health. Coconut oil contains a large quantity of beneficial constituents that have been the subject of a great deal of current scientific research.

This valuable oil is obtained through both "wet" and "dry" processes. The dry process extracts the oil from crushed and air-dried coconut meat, known as *copra,* which is pressed or dissolved with solvents (such as hexane), producing the coconut oil and a high-protein, high-fiber mash that is unfit for human consumption but is instead used as animal feed. The wet process uses raw coconuts to produce an emulsion of oil and water. To recover the oil, modern techniques use cen-trifuges and pretreatments, including cold, heat, acids, salts, enzymes, electrolysis, shock waves, or some combination of them. Virgin coconut oil can be produced from fresh coco-nut milk, meat, or residue. Producing it from the fresh meat involves removing the shell, washing the meat, and then either wet-milling or drying it and using a screw press to extract the oil. Virgin coconut oil has a white to yellowish color and an aroma like that of fresh coconut.

At room temperature, coconut oil forms a solid. Only when it is warmed up to 86°F (30°C) does it begin to melt and become fluid. Coconut oil is very heat-resistant, mak-ing it well suited for cooking. Depending on the manner in which it was produced, its smoke point lies between about

Tips for Using Coconut Oil

If the coconut oil you wish to use for oil pulling or for external use is solid, you should heat it only enough to melt it. One simple way to do so is to use a spoon to place a small amount into a bowl, which you can then place directly in the sun or on a heater (never directly on a flame). Another easy method is to heat the coconut oil in a water bath: Place approximately two tablespoons of coconut oil in a tall, small container. Place this into another container that has been half-filled with water. Then warm the water carefully and slowly. Under no circumstances should you warm the oil in a microwave oven, for the microwaves will alter the molecular makeup of the oil and impair its positive effects.

350 and 400°F (177°C and 204°C), and its burning point is around 536°F (280°C). As coconut oil melts, it absorbs heat from its surroundings. This can produce a distinct sensation of cooling in the mouth. For this reason, coconut oil is used in the manufacture of many popular frozen confections.

Storage and Shelf Life

Thanks to its high content of saturated fats, coconut oil enjoys a comparably long shelf life, allowing it to be stored without problems for up to two years. An additional advantage is that coconut oil does not need to be kept cool. Coconut oil can be stored wherever one has room, although a relatively dark and dry location is preferable.

Effects

Coconut oil contains over 90 percent saturated fats, predominantly short- and medium-chain triglycerides. The most prevalent of these is lauric acid (52 percent); the most common monounsaturated fatty acid is oleic acid (8 percent). Coconut oil also contains polyphenols, and it is these secondary plant substances that give coconut oil its aroma and taste. Also present are high amounts of vitamins E and K, as well as iron and organic sulfur. Because of the saturated fats found in coconut oil, it has long been used as an edible fat and oil.

Over the years, there has been considerable debate about the health benefits of coconut oil. Part of the confusion is due to the fact that the coconut oil used some years ago had been subjected to a great deal of processing that removed or changed the healthy constituents in the oil. In addition, the large quantities of lauric acid were thought to have harmful effects. However, recent scientific studies have shown that lauric acid contributes to the normalization of body fat values and also has anti-inflammatory as well as antibacterial, antiviral, and antifungal effects. Lauric acid is now considered beneficial to our health.

Because of its positive effects on blood lipid levels, lauric acid is different from other saturated fatty acids. Ingesting lauric acid does not lead to an increase in LDL "bad" cholesterol levels but instead helps protect the heart. By preventing harm to the arterial walls and thus the development of atherosclerosis, lauric acid can also help treat high blood pressure. Coconut oil fortifies the digestive system and improves the intake of such important vital substances as vitamins, minerals, and amino acids through the digestive tract and into the body. Since coconut oil is easily digestible, it boosts the metabolism, so that a large number of calories are consumed as it is broken down. Hence, coconut oil can also help in losing weight. Coconut oil also promotes healthy skin and hair. Its strong moisturizing effects help keep the skin from drying out and also prevent the accumulation of fats. Coconut oil can contribute to healthy, fast hair growth, and the proteins present in the oil can help regenerate damaged hair. This makes coconut oil ideal for deep conditioning.

Flaxseed Oil

Flaxseed oil is obtained from the ripe seeds of the flax plant (*Linum usitatissimum*). This culturally important plant was already highly regarded in the time of the ancient Egyptians. Flaxseed oil can be used for many purposes. In addition to its use in the kitchen and in health care, it is also used in the manufacture of varnishes, oil paints, linoleum, and even soap. For these industrial purposes the oil is extracted with heat and solvents and called linseed oil. It is also used as a preservative treatment for wood.

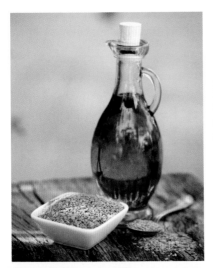

Depending on whether flaxseed oil is obtained through cold or warm pressing, it can be used for culinary, medicinal, or technical purposes.

High-quality flaxseed oil for culinary use is obtained through cold pressing. The oil is pressed out of prepared flax-seeds with a screw press. In this way it is exposed to only low pressure and kept at a temperature below 104°F (40°C). The oil produced in this fashion possesses the characteristic dark golden color and typical clean, mild, nutty aroma of flaxseeds, and in this way the valuable constituents found in the oil are preserved.

Storage and Shelf Life

Flaxseed oil can quickly turn bitter and rancid. For this reason it should be stored in a dark, cool space or in the refrigerator. As well, the oil is best kept in a dark-colored bottle. Once the bottle has been opened, the oil should be used within three weeks. Flaxseed oil has a very low melting point of approximately −4 to 3°F (−20 to −16°C), so that it can be stored in the freezer compartment without solidifying. Doing so will prevent spoilage for several additional weeks.

Effects

Flaxseed oil contains 72 percent polyunsaturated fatty acids consisting of approximately 13 percent linoleic acid and 58 percent linolenic acid. As little as 40 to 50 grams of flax-seed oil is sufficient to meet our daily requirement of these valuable unsaturated fatty acids. Flaxseed oil also contains high amounts of vitamins A and E, as well as lecithin and lignans, phytoestrogens with antioxidant effects. These substances can help reduce the risk of heart attack, and they lower LDL cholesterol levels in the blood. Flaxseed oil also helps reduce high blood pressure, strengthens the immune

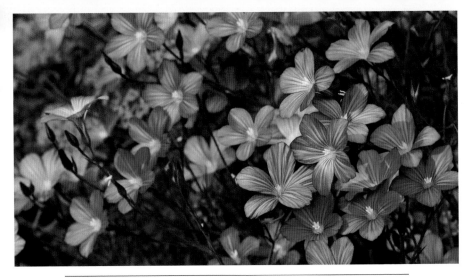

The flax plant can grow up to 2 and ½ feet (70 cm) tall.
The blue blooms develop into round capsules containing brown seeds.

system, and provides relief for rheumatic illnesses. It is recommended that flaxseed oil be added to quark, a type of fresh, unripened cheese, because the sulfur-containing amino acids present in the quark improve the solubility of the fatty acids and facilitate their absorption by the body.

Olive Oil

Olive oil, sometimes called "green gold," is considered among the oils that are the best for our health. Produced from the flesh of olive fruits, it has been regarded as an elixir of health in the Mediterranean region for millennia. Even the ancient Egyptians, including the pharaoh Ramses II, who reached the astonishing (for that time) age of sixty-four years, ingested olive oil for all types of ailments.

The best olive oil, which is produced by cold-pressing the highest-quality olives, is referred to as *extra virgin*. It has been produced in essentially the same manner for centuries, though today's technology can do this both more rapidly and more hygienically. After harvesting, the olives are immediately washed and separated from the stems and leaves. The entire fruit, including the pit, oil, and juice, is ground and reduced to a soft mass. In traditional presses, the olive mass is spread onto woven mats that are placed on one another and then hydraulically pressed. The resulting mixture of water and oil is channeled into a catch basin, where the lighter oil naturally separates out and collects at the water's surface. Today, both the pressing process and the separation of water and oil are increasingly performed with the help of centrifuges. This requires less time than traditional methods of pressing, allowing more oil to be produced in a shorter amount of time. No matter how the olive oil is produced, it is important that the temperature not exceed 81°F (27°C). It is only through such cold pressing that the valuable but heat-sensitive substances are preserved in the oil.

Storage and Shelf Life

Because of the composition of its fatty acids, olive oil will stay fresh much longer than many other types of plant oil. When stored in a dark, cool location and maintained at a temperature between 50 and 60°F (10 and 16°C), an unopened bottle of olive oil can remain unspoiled for up to twelve months. Once opened, the contents of a bottle should be used within two months. When olive oil is stored in the refrigerator, the oil may flocculate, causing whitish particles to appear. These do not affect the quality of the oil and will disappear when the oil is rewarmed, preferable in sunlight or warm water.

🌿

The Three Grades of Olive Oil

European Union guidelines distinguish between three grades of olive oil. The determining factor is the content of free fatty acids, which provides an unambiguous indication of the level of quality and therewith the grade to which a particular olive oil will be assigned. The lower the percentage of fatty acids found in the oil, the higher its grade. Producers in Italy, Greece, and Spain (all members of the European Union) use this system to grade their oils.

The first and best grade includes oils that are considered to be perfect in taste, aroma, and color. In addition, the oil must be obtained in such a manner that it cannot be altered, as when, for example, the oil is processed with solvents. Also, oils of this highest quality may not be subjected to any processes other than washing, filtration, and centrifugation, and the maximum acid content cannot exceed 1 to 2 percent. If all of these criteria are met, the oil is designated as **native olive oil** (from the Latin *nativus,* "indigenous" or "natural"). The second quality grade is referred to as **refined olive oil** (*Olio di oliva raffinato* or *Huile d'olive faffinée*). This is obtained by refining native olive oils using heat, a process that alters the oil. The third grade recognized by the European Union classification system is comprised of olive oils whose high acid content adversely affects their taste and aroma. Native oil is added to these to impart the typical olive oil aroma. This blend is sold under the label **olive oil**.

When possible, only native olive oil should be used for oil pulling; the second and third quality grades should be avoided. A further distinction is made between two types of native olive oil. The first is **extra virgin olive oil.** These four words guarantee that you are using a high-quality, naturally pure olive oil with a perfect taste that has been obtained through cold pressing; it is unrefined and free of chemical additives. Only such oil can be referred to as "extra virgin" (*Olio extra vergine di oliva* in Italian and *Huile d'olive vierge extra* in French). To be classified as extra virgin, the fatty-acid content may not exceed one gram per hundred grams. The second type of native olive oil is called **virgin olive oil.** If the acid content does exceed the I percent mark, then the oil may only be marketed as virgin olive oil. This oil (*Olio vergine di oliva* in Italian and *Huile d'olive vierge* in French) may not contain more than two grams of free fatty acids for every hundred grams of oil.

Effects

According to current scientific understanding, olive oil is one of the very best oils for our health. It contains a high content of vitamin E and up to 80 percent monounsaturated oleic acid. The remainder includes diunsaturated and saturated fatty acids. This unique constellation of fatty acids has a very positive effect on our health. Some of the benefits of olive oil include lowering harmful LDL cholesterol and excessively high blood pressure, thereby protecting the heart and blood vessels. In countries in which large amounts of olive oil are part of the traditional diet, as in the Mediterranean region, the rates of cardiovascular disease are significantly lower than in countries where little olive oil is used. Because olive oil is rich in antioxidants, substances that protect the cells from the effects of free radicals, consuming it can also help prevent certain types of cancers.

Peanut Oil

The oil obtained from the oil-rich seeds of the peanut plant (*Arachis hypogaea*) has a long history of use in Asian cuisine. Because peanut oil has a high smoke point—somewhere around 446°F (230°C)—it is well suited for such high-temperature cooking procedures as broiling, simmering, grilling, and frying. Because of its healthy ingredients and its multifaceted uses, peanut oil has recently been winning fans outside of Asia and has found uses outside the kitchen—for example, as a skin-care agent and in oil pulling.

Peanuts are legumes and not true nuts. Once the seeds have been shelled and dried, the manufacture of the oil occurs in a screw press. Cold-pressed peanut oil is produced without the use of any external heat source, including roasting or treating with steam. After pressing, the oil is filtered but not refined. In this way, most of the beneficial constituents are

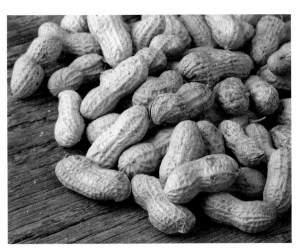

One important advantage of peanut oil is its long shelf life. Compared to other oils, peanut oil does not easily turn rancid.

retained. High-quality peanut oil has a yellowish color and a strong, nutty taste.

Storage and Shelf Life

Like many plant oils, peanut oil is sensitive to light, oxygen, and heat and should thus be stored in a cold, dark place. Once opened, the bottle should always be closed tightly after each use. Depending on the type, peanut oil can be stored in its original, unopened container for up to twenty-four months. When peanut oil is exposed to temperatures below 50°F (10°C), it gels and becomes viscous, and it solidifies between 33 and 38°F (1 and 3°C). Gently warming the oil, however, will return it to its original consistency. This should not be done directly over a flame but rather by submerging the oil in some hot (not boiling) water.

Effects

Peanut oil possesses high amounts of vitamin E: 100 grams of peanut oil contain approximately 23 milligrams. Peanut oil also contains relatively high amounts of vitamin B_1, D, and K. The fatty-acid component of peanut oil consists of approximately 44 percent polyunsaturated fatty acids (primarily linoleic acid), 37 percent monounsaturated fatty acids (chiefly oleic acid), and around 20 percent saturated fats. Peanut oil helps regulate high blood pressure, and it lowers the levels of LDL cholesterol and triglycerides in the blood. Because of its high vitamin E content, peanut oil also strengthens the body's immune processes and promotes cell renewal. Due to its relaxing effects, peanut oil is also becoming a popular bath as well as massage oil.

Pumpkin Seed Oil

Pumpkin seed oil is produced from the roasted seeds of the Styrian oil pumpkin (*Cucurbita pepo* var. *styriaca*). It is a culinary specialty from what had formerly been part of the Kingdom of Hungary and is presently southeastern Austria (Styria), eastern Slovenia (Styria and Prekmurje), central Transylvania, the Orastie-Cugir region of Romania, northwestern Croatia, and adjacent regions of Hungary. It is a European Union Protected Designation of Origin (PDO) product. This variety of pumpkin is different from other pumpkins in that its seeds are nonwoody. Only a fine, silvery skin protects the soft seed, from which the uniquely excellent pumpkin seed oil is pressed.

Genuine Styrian pumpkin seed oil is produced under continuous oversight, is marked with a seal of quality, and is labeled *100 percent Pure Pumpkin Seed Oil*. European Union regulations stipulate that this name can only be used for products made in a specific geographic region. Due to the elaborate steps involved in its manufacture, high-quality pumpkin seed oil is one of the most prized and expensive of oils. For this reason, and because of its shiny, petroleum-like appearance, pumpkin seed oil is often referred to as "Styrian black gold."

Manufacturing pumpkin seed oil is a relatively complex process that entails a number of steps. After the pulp and the seeds have been separated, the seeds are freed from the remains of the husk and then washed. Afterward, the seeds are dried, thereby reducing their water content to just 8 percent. This makes it easier to store and handle the seeds. The next step involves grinding the seeds. To be able to extract the oil, the resulting ground, dried mass of seeds is mixed with

The Black Gold of the Kitchen

Although its low smoke point of 248°F (120°C) means that pumpkin seed oil is poorly suited for grilling or frying, it nevertheless deserves a place in the kitchen, for apart from its healthy effects it is also a treat for the palate. Its characteristically intense nutty aroma and flavor add a delicate note to tomatoes, sauces, soups, and egg and meat dishes. Pumpkin seed oil serves as an excellent salad dressing when combined with honey or olive oil, while the typical Styrian dressing consists of pumpkin seed oil and apple cider vinegar. Pumpkin seed oil is also an excellent complement to both hard and fresh cheeses and can even be used as a topping for vanilla ice cream. Using it as a cooking oil, however, destroys its essential fatty acids and this is to be avoided.

water and salt. The mixture is then heated to around 112°F (50°C). At this temperature, the mass is stirred constantly as it is carefully roasted. This causes the water to evaporate, at which time the unmistakable aroma of the pumpkin seed oil—an intense nutty fragrance—develops. The mass is then pressed in an oil mill, yielding the viscous, dark green oil. The remaining solids settle in about a week or are separated through filtration.

Storage and Shelf Life

Thanks to the special ways in which the pumpkin seeds are treated, they can be stored for some time, allowing the manufacturer to press and sell pumpkin seed oil throughout the year as needed. This oil is more sensitive to light than other oils and must consequently always be stored in a dark, cool place. For this reason, pumpkin seed oil is usually packaged in relatively small, dark-colored bottles that can be quickly consumed. Once opened, a bottle of pumpkin seed oil should be kept in the refrigerator and used quickly. In contrast, an unopened bottle of pumpkin seed oil can be stored for up to nine months.

Effects

Pumpkin seed oil has a high content of mono- and polyunsaturated fatty acids, including oleic and linoleic acids. It also contains significant amounts of vitamins A, B, C, D, and E, protein, and minerals such as calcium, phosphorus, and magnesium. Also present are the trace elements iron, selenium, and zinc. These large amounts of health-promoting substances help lower LDL cholesterol and triglyceride levels, lower blood pressure, and regulate the metabolism. Easily digestible, pumpkin seed oil is often used in folk medicine to treat bladder infections, irritable bladder, and prostate ailments.

Safflower Oil

This oil is obtained from the ripe seeds of the safflower (*Carthamus tinctorius*). The safflower is a very old cultural plant that was cultivated in Egypt as long ago as 3500 BC. The botanical species name *tinctorius* refers to its use as a dye for coloring linen garments and textiles. The safflower was brought to Europe during the Middle Ages, and it remains a popular garden plant because of its bright yellow-orange petals.

High-quality safflower oil is obtained through cold pressing. The lower-quality varieties are either refined or extracted,

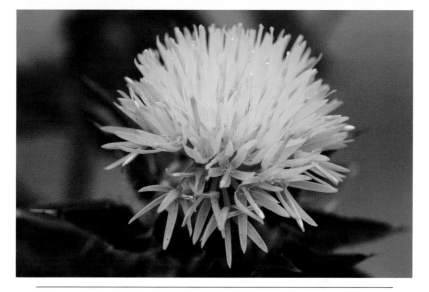

Safflower oil is used in cooking as well as cosmetics and medicine.

and their production typically involves high temperatures. In addition, the lower-quality varieties of safflower oil are often treated with chemicals to increase their shelf life. These procedures rob the oil of a large part of its beneficial ingredients. In contrast, cold pressing is much gentler because it occurs at much lower temperatures, thereby ensuring that the beneficial substances remain in the oil. Safflower oil obtained through cold pressing has a strong, zesty taste of its own, whereas the refined oil is almost tasteless. This is one way that you can tell whether you have purchased a high-quality oil.

Storage and Shelf Life

When stored in a dark, cool, well-sealed location, safflower oil will remain fresh for some nine to twelve months. It is important to note that safflower oil can quickly spoil if exposed to oxygen or sunlight. To protect it from exposure to light, safflower oil should be stored in dark glass bottles. An opened bottle should be stored away from windows and heat sources such as a stove.

Effects

Of all plant oils, safflower oil possesses the greatest amount of diunsaturated linoleic acid; a good safflower oil may contain up to 78 percent. The remainder consists of monounsaturated and a maximum of 10 percent saturated fatty acids. The oil also contains high amounts of vitamins A, E, and K. Safflower oil lowers LDL cholesterol and triglyceride levels, thereby providing protection against cardiovascular illnesses and atherosclerosis (the accumulation of plaque on the inside walls of the arteries). It also strengthens the immune system, promotes cell renewal, and has anti-inflammatory effects. For this reason it is often used in cosmetics to treat skin problems. It is also used as a massage oil.

Sesame Oil

Sesame oil is obtained from the seeds of *Sesamum indicum,* a member of the Pedaliaceae or sesame family. Sesame is one of humankind's oldest cultigens and has been esteemed as a source of oil since ancient times. A distinction is made

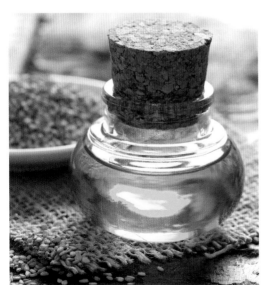

Sesame is originally from Africa and India.

between light and dark sesame seed oil; whereas the light oil is made from untreated sesame seeds, dark sesame seed oil is produced by briefly roasted the seeds before pressing. This imparts a deep, rich color and a piquant taste to the oil.

Storage and Shelf Life

In comparison to other plant oils, sesame oil may be stored for very long periods of time; unopened, it will remain fresh for twelve months or more. Once opened, however, the contents of a bottle should be used within three months.

Effects

Sesame seed oil contains a healthy combination of fatty acids and is also rich in minerals, trace elements, and lecithin. It can improve heart function, reduce harmful cholesterol, help prevent osteoporosis, and strengthen the bones and teeth. In ayurveda, sesame oil plays a central role in many treatments, and it is ideal for treating dry and flaky skin, making it well suited for use as a massage oil.

Sunflower Oil

The sunflower (*Helianthus annuus*) is not only pretty to look at, its hard seeds are the source of a valuable oil. The oil is obtained by cleaning, drying, and—depending on the type of sunflower—shelling the seeds before pressing. The processing of unshelled or partially shelled seeds yields an oil with a dark yellow color and a very pronounced taste. Cold-pressed sunflower oil is produced in small oil mills using screw presses. This gentle process ensures that the valuable vitamins and fatty acids are retained.

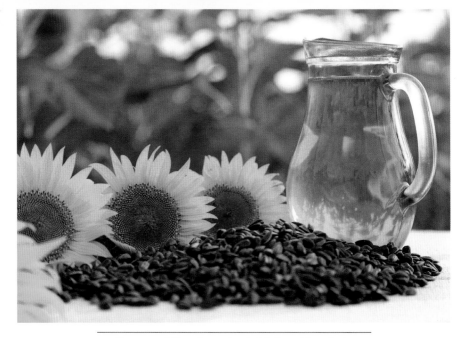

Because of its polyunsaturated fatty acid content,
sunflower oil is one of our most valuable oils.

Storage and Shelf Life

Sunflower oil is very light-sensitive and should therefore be stored in a cool, dark place. In its original sealed bottle, the oil has a shelf life of up to a year. Once a container has been opened, however, it should be stored in the refrigerator.

Effects

Sunflower oil has a high content—65 percent—of polyunsaturated fatty acids. It is also a good source of magnesium and calcium, the trace elements phosphorus, silicon, and fluorine, and vitamins B, D, and E. Sunflower oil contains more vitamin D than cod liver oil and more B vitamins than wheat germ oil (see facing page). The oil lowers the content of LDL "bad" cholesterol, prevents heart and circulatory aliments, and helps in cases of constipation.

Wheat Germ Oil

The germ of the ancient cultigen wheat (*Triticum vulgare*) is the source of one of our most expensive plant oils. Its high price is a result of the relatively low yield of this grain: 1,600 kilograms of wheat are needed to obtain just one liter of wheat germ oil. The golden yellow oil is manufactured through a very gentle form of cold pressing, ensuring that the oil remains lukewarm throughout the process.

Storage and Shelf Life

Like almost all plant oils, wheat germ oil should be protected from light and stored in a cool place. When left in an unopened bottle, the oil has a shelf life of up to a year. Once opened, however, wheat germ oil should be stored in the refrigerator, and the contents of a bottle should be used within six to eight weeks.

Effects

Wheat germ oil has a very high content—64 percent—of polyunsaturated fatty acids, primarily linoleic and linolenic acids. The amounts of vitamin E and magnesium are impressive: as little as one tablespoon of wheat germ oil provides the daily vitamin E requirement of an adult, while four tablespoons of pure wheat germ oil contain half the daily requirement of magnesium. Wheat germ oil helps strengthen the immune system, regulates fat metabolism, and protects against cardiovascular ailments.

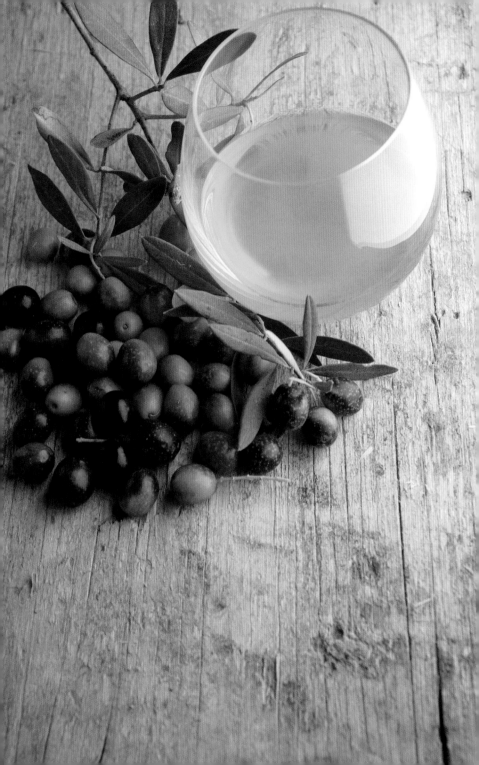

Complementary Detoxification Techniques

The practice of oil pulling can be wonderfully supported by using additional, complementary methods to purify and detoxify the body. Like oil pulling, some of these can easily be incorporated into your daily routine. Others can be practiced at regular intervals as part of a health-maintenance regime. The two most important factors in keeping the body free of toxins are a healthy diet and regular physical activity, which stimulates the metabolism and circulation.

The Importance of Good Dietary Habits

Proper nutrition can contribute enormously to freeing the body from metabolic wastes, toxins, and other harmful substances. This can be accomplished by focusing on those foods known to detoxify and unburden the body. Such foods are almost exclusively alkaline-forming (as opposed to

Your Daily Regimen

To promote and maintain health, it is important to:

- Drink two to three liters of still (noncarbonated) water and herbal tea daily
- Eat a diet rich in fiber
- Receive adequate supplies of vitamins, minerals, and other needed substances
- Have ample physical activity
- Avoid negative stress as much as possible

acid-forming). To promote the elimination of waste products and other harmful substances, a rule of thumb is to eat as much alkaline-forming food as possible, by consuming at least twice as much as acid-forming food.

The Acid-Alkaline Balance

Excess acid in the body is harmful on every level, yet most of us consume an excess of acid-forming foods. This brings our sensitive acid-alkaline balance out of equilibrium, with many negative consequences. Acidity can weaken our immune mechanisms and cause chronic pain in the joints and intervertebral disks, such that you hurt all over. Frequent headaches, fatigue, and poor concentration can also result from an overabundance of acid in the body. A persistently acidic diet can also affect our physical appearance by contributing to skin afflictions, wrinkling, and other signs of aging and a weakening of connective tissues.

Normally, wastes, toxins, and other harmful substances are systematically metabolized, but this natural regulation can be impaired by excess acidity. Instead of eliminating acidic residues, the body stores them, which leads to an accumulation of waste products in the body. An excessively acid condition inhibits the excretion of waste products, toxins, and other harmful substances and thus is one of the main causes of the previously mentioned ailments.

What can you do to prevent this harmful overacidification? You should eat an abundance of alkaline-forming foods and reduce or omit acid-forming foods from your diet. Like a spring cleaning, this will help relieve and revitalize your body and give you renewed energy. It will also help prevent your body from even beginning to store an overabundance of waste products. Nutrition experts recommend consuming a balance of 70 percent alkaline to 30 percent acidic foods throughout the day. In other words, we should nourish ourselves with approximately twice the amount of alkaline-forming foods as acid-forming foods. This two-to-one formula is not to be followed slavishly; if the proportion of alkaline-builders to acid-builders does not have the proper balance on one day, you can easily adjust it the next by favoring alkaline foods. These guidelines also do not mean that you should *never* eat acid-forming foods again. A balanced and healthy nutrition includes both alkaline and acid foods; they should simply be eaten in the proper ratio.

Restoring Your Acid-Alkaline Balance

What is alkaline and what is acidic? Which foods help form alkaline compounds and may therefore be called alkaline-builders? Which form acids and are called acid-builders?

Simplified considerably, as a kind of an overall snapshot,

Alkaline-Building Foods

- Still (noncarbonated) mineral water
- Herbal teas
- Most vegetable varieties (for the exceptions, see the acid-builders)
- Mushrooms
- Sprouts
- Vegetable broths
- Fresh herbs (except for cress)
- Most fruits, especially bananas and coconut (for the exceptions, see the acid-builders)
- Dried fruits
- Pear juice
- Raw milk
- Whey
- Raw milk cream
- Raw milk butter
- Soy products
- Olive oil
- Seafood

we can say that all animal products are acid-builders. In addition to all meats and fish, this list includes eggs and milk products (except for unpasteurized raw milk products, which are alkaline), alcohol, and coffee. Most nuts and grains are also acid-builders, as are most oils. In contrast, alkaline-builders include many (but not all) vegetables, fruits, and fresh herbs and such protein sources as almonds, tempeh, and tofu. Their metabolic breakdown produces many alkaline compounds that bind to excessive free acids, thereby helping to restore the acid-alkaline balance. The chart that follows lists many of the common alkaline-builders and acid-builders.

Acid-Building Foods

- Alcoholic beverages (wine, beer, etc.)
- Some vegetables: artichokes, Brussels sprouts, asparagus, spinach, winter squash, corn
- All grains (except millet)
- Legumes
- Unripe fruits
- Some produce, such as citrus fruits and rhubarb
- All nuts (except for almonds and walnuts)
- Sugar
- Sweets of any type
- Cheese (pasteurized)
- Quark (fresh non-aged cheese)
- Eggs
- Meat, fish, and poultry
- Meat broths

Foods That Detoxify

Some foods are especially well suited for purging toxins from the body. Among those that are especially useful are pineapple, kiwi, mango, and papaya. These fruits contain many enzymes that provide intensive stimulation to the metabolism and promote digestion. As a bonus, they also help detoxify the digestive tract. Other foods that you should eat frequently include bilberries, raspberries, strawberries, and melons, the last of which also help the body expel excess water.

Bitter vegetables, especially chicory and arugula, can also be used to kick-start the detoxification process. These promote the functioning of the liver and gallbladder, thereby producing additional detoxifying effects. Other recommended detoxifiers are broccoli, bell peppers, red beets, fennel, zucchini, and carrots. Another food item that is ideal for detoxification and

Bromelain, a Useful Supplement for Alkalizing the Body

Due to dietary and other factors, most of us are way too acidic, in which case taking a supplement of bromelain—particularly when the preponderance of foods we eat tend to be acidic—can help restore the proper acid-alkaline balance, assist in digestion, and remove that puffy or full feeling that can result from too acid a condition. Bromelain is a protein extract derived from the stems of pineapples, although it exists in all parts of the fresh plant and fruit. Pineapples have a long tradition as a medicinal plant among the natives of South and Central America. The first isolation of bromelain was recorded by the Venezuelan chemist Vicente Marcano in 1891, through fermentation of the fruit of pineapple. Later, the term *bromelain* was introduced and applied to any protease from any member of the plant family Bromeliaceae. Bromelain is widely available in health food stores and online vitamin retailers.

promoting the excretion of excess water is rice. This is why some detoxification regimens are based on the use of rice (see the next section on giving your body a time-out). It is also important to drink adequate amounts of fresh, noncarbonated water daily. Noncarbonated "still" water tops the list of detoxifying and alkaline-building items that are essential in your diet. To further promote detoxification, one suggestion is to abstain from eating fresh fruits and raw vegetables after 2 p.m. to avoid overstimulating the digestive processes.

Give Your Body a Time-Out

One wonderful way to give your digestive system a break and free your body of waste products and toxins is to go on a kind of semifast for two or three days each month. On these days consume only fresh water, vegetable and fruit juices, and either fruit or rice. During these days you should abstain from such items as coffee, black tea, and of course alcohol, all of which hinder detoxification and counteract your efforts. During these "time-out" days you should also abstain from salt. Salt binds water in our bodies, making it more difficult to expel waste products. Another ideal step for detoxifying and purging the body of excess water is to eat two to three fresh pineapples by themselves (i.e., without sweeteners, cream, or other additives) throughout the day. Consumed on a regular basis (the rich flavor makes this no problem at all), pineapple contains an enzyme that stimulates protein digestion and promotes the excretion of metabolic toxins and excess water as well as the shedding of unwanted pounds. Another method well suited to purging the body of waste products is to have some days on which all you eat is boiled rice. More on fasting—when and how—can be found later in this book.

Detoxify with Delight

As we have seen, there are many ways we can "take out the trash" in our bodies by simply adjusting what we eat. Another effective and efficient way is through any number of detoxification regimens. The word *detoxify* means to remove poisons from the body, and this is what we are doing when we clean out the body. That the simplest things are often the best should not surprise us, least of all when we are talking about the foods we

Artichoke: The Healthy Finger Food

The flower of the artichoke plant—a type of thistle— can be simply boiled in water to make a magnificent appetizer. You will not need your knife or fork for this dish, as you can remove the leaves with your fingers and dip them into different types of spicy sauces. This finger food is as healthy as can be and is perfect for those who are working on losing weight: with just 91 calories per 100 grams, the artichoke is a true lightweight. It is also highly recommended for diabetics because the starch found in the artichoke, known as *inulin,* does not affect blood sugar.

Before boiling, break or cut the stem directly below the flower (you can usually buy artichokes with the stem already removed). Remove the lowest three or four hard, fibrous leaves as well. Use kitchen shears to cut off the thorny points of the remaining leaves. Cover the entire artichoke with water and then boil for at least thirty minutes with a pinch of salt and some lemon juice. The artichoke is ready to serve when you are able to gently pull out the leaves. Place artichoke on a serving plate and enjoy this healthy feast! Holding the tip of the leaf (the end from which you cut the thorn) between your thumb and forefinger, place the leaf between your teeth, close your mouth, and then pull on the leaf. Your front teeth will strip the meaty flesh off the leaf. As you continue working your way to the center, or heart, of the artichoke, the leaves will become increasingly tender.

After you have finished eating the leaves, scrape off the fibers that adhere to the heart and discard them. Now you can enjoy the tender heart of the artichoke flower, which most people consider to be its best part.

ingest every day. Natural, unprocessed foods should be free of additional ingredients, flavor enhancers, and coloring agents. The basic principle of detoxifying is that by eating such foods we are assisting the body in ridding itself of its accumulated toxins and other harmful substances.

Taking Out the Trash

The process of detoxifying helps the liver and kidneys eliminate waste such as urea, uric acid, and sulfur that collects in the body. Eliminating this "trash" helps restore our energy level and zest for life and helps us regain vitality and a sense of contentment. It enhances our body awareness and helps pay better attention to the needs of our body. By eating more consciously and in moderation, by consuming smaller amounts of animal fats, proteins, and sugar, by drinking herbal teas instead of coffee, and by eating more rice and vegetables in place of fried meats—even if only for a few days a week—we can help our body stay in a better state of balance. This also frees our mind, for detoxifying is not only about developing healthier eating habits, it is also about clearing our mind. This is why an important part of any detoxification program involves positive thinking. Metabolic wastes and toxins represent more than just the crude wastes produced by the digestive processes; they are also the trash of our mental attitudes.

The Concept of Detoxification

Is detoxification about sacrifice, fasting, or calorie counting? Not at all. Detoxifying has less to do with weight loss and more to do with feeling well. In fact, the goal of detoxification is not to lose weight, but to gain in physical awareness, vitality, and zest for life.

When detoxifying, it is necessary to abstain from all those things that place an unnecessary burden on your body—specifically, prepackaged and fast foods, breaded and fried foods, sweets and sugar substitutes, and saturated fats. Other taboos include products made with bleached wheat flour, white sugar, alcohol, and nicotine. And last but certainly not least, to help yourself remember how to consciously enjoy things with all your senses, try turning off your television, radio, computer, and cell phone for periods of time while you are detoxifying.

What Does Belong on the Table?

To facilitate the body's normal detoxification process, what are the foods that we should eat and what are the ones we should avoid? Here are seven golden rules:

The First Rule of Detoxifying

Eat: seafood, such as halibut and salmon, which are rich in beneficial omega-3 fats

Avoid: beef, pork, lamb, and poultry

The Second Rule of Detoxifying

Eat: natural sweets such as honey and maple syrup (in moderation) and stevia

Avoid: refined white sugar, high-fructose corn syrup, and
artificial sweeteners

The Third Rule of Detoxifying

Eat: aromatic herbs and spices that promote digestion, such
as basil, cumin, rosemary, and ginger
Avoid: packaged soups and sauces, mustard, ketchup,
mayonnaise, and soy sauce

The Fourth Rule of Detoxifying

Eat: natural grains high in fiber, such as wild rice,
buckwheat, oats, and amaranth (these should be unrefined
and not consumed in the form of bread or baked goods)
Avoid: wheat, rye, bleached wheat flour products,
prepackaged muesli, cornflakes, crackers, and cookies

The Fifth Rule of Detoxifying

Eat: cold-pressed plant oils, such as sesame, sunflower, and olive
Avoid: saturated and animal fats as well as refined oils

The Sixth Rule of Detoxifying

Eat: unroasted, unsalted nuts and seeds, such as almonds,
walnuts, pumpkin seeds, and sunflower seeds, and
legumes such as beans, lentils, and chickpeas
Avoid: such protein sources as pasteurized milk products,
soy products, and eggs

The Seventh Rule of Detoxifying

Eat: green, leafy vegetables that are rich in antioxidants,
such as spinach, green cabbage, and kale, as well as other
colored vegetables such as beets, squash, and carrots
Avoid: nightshades—potatoes, tomatoes, peppers, and eggplant

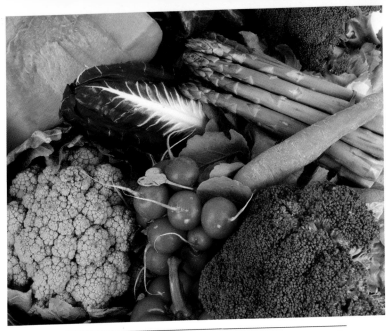

Detoxifying means cleansing with delight. Avoid potatoes and tomatoes and eat lots of leafy vegetables.

Care of the Lips

The skin of the lips is especially tender and thus requires special care. Because your lips do not contain any oil glands it is recommended that you regularly treat them with jojoba oil or cocoa butter. Coconut oil also makes a good lip balm. You can also use these oils and fatty substances to massage the areas directly above and below your lips. This helps protect these areas from wrinkles and will help keep your lips from becoming dry and cracked. Especially when it is cold or you have been exposed to excessive sun or salt water, such as when you are on vacation, you should ensure that your lips retain their moisture.

Your Seven-Day Detoxification Plan

First Day: "Clear the Decks"

Your short vacation from your regular nutritional grind begins today. Your diet for the next seven days will allow your body to take a break. On this first day and over the next six days, the following rules apply:

- Drink eight glasses of fresh water daily.
- Avoid coffee, tea, and other caffeinated beverages.
- Abstain from alcohol and nicotine.
- Avoid all carbonated beverages.
- Instead of refined sugars or artificial sweeteners, enhance your meals with honey, maple syrup, or stevia.
- Avoid refined white flour products.
- Avoid meat and poultry. Instead, eat fish such as wild salmon or halibut, as well as legumes, seeds, sprouts, and unsalted, unroasted nuts.
- Make sure that your food comes from certified organic sources.

Second Day: "Power Food"

Now that you have removed the most important food "sins" from your menu, it is time to turn to the foods that will help you rebuild. On this day it is especially important that you drink a lot of fresh water and eat nuts from time to time to maintain your energy level.

- Eat a lot of colored vegetables, such as squash, carrots, and beets, as well as leafy greens and salads.
- Avoid nightshades, including tomatoes, potatoes, peppers, and eggplants.

➤ Eat a lot of fresh fruit (however, citrus, dried fruits, and preserved fruits are taboo).

➤ Season your meals with fresh herbs.

Third Day: "Milk Break"

➤ Today, leave out all milk and milk products. Use almond or rice milk instead.*

➤ Avoid both egg and soy products.

➤ Add pumpkin or sunflower seeds to your meals.

➤ Between meals eat a handful of unsalted and unroasted nuts.

➤ For delicious between-meal snacks, eat apple slices with a dab of nut butter, carrot sticks, or chilled grapes.

Fourth Day: "Good Grains"

The last course correction for your plate involves using natural, unprocessed grains. In addition, concentrate intensely on the detoxification process. Doing so will provide mental support for your body's cleanup work.

➤ Avoid products made of corn (i.e., tortilla chips) and wheat, as well as baked goods and baked sweets.

➤ Eat amaranth, natural and wild rice, buckwheat, millet, or oats.

➤ Use olive, sesame, and sunflower oils.

---

*Read the package label carefully when buying commercial almond or rice milk; many products include soy milk along with unnatural "flavor enhancers." Easy instructions for making your own rice or almond milk are readily available online.

Fifth Day: "Coming Down"

The motto of the next two days is to spoil yourself in every way. It takes energy for your body to clean itself up. While you are undertaking this cure, the energy your metabolic processes are using will not be available for other things. Take the opportunity to slow down, reflect, and focus on your inner self.

- Do you feel like having some chocolate or a cup of coffee? Reward yourself instead with some gentle exercise, like going for a walk or doing some yoga. Afterward you will find that your cravings have disappeared.

Sixth Day: "Indulge"

On this day, indulge yourself with a day of comprehensive care. Here are a few ideas:

- Take a warm shower and have a full body scrub, for example with sea salt. Following a circular motion, massage the salt into your wet skin and then shower it away. Finish up by applying a rich, moisturizing oil.
- Allow someone else to massage you.
- A facial steam bath can help support your skin during the purification process. Add a few drops of eucalyptus oil or simply place a teaspoon of chamomile into a bowl of hot water. Position your face over the bowl, place a towel over your head, and allow the purifying steam to work its magic for ten minutes. Afterward, dry your face and avoid the fresh air for half an hour.

On this, the last day of your detoxification, ask yourself: "How do I feel?" Do you want to resume your normal eating habits or continue with this detoxifying regimen? No matter what you decide, notice how strong you feel both physically and emotionally. Perhaps you will decide to make detoxifying a part of your regular health-maintenance program.

- If you do decide to resume your old eating habits, do so gradually. Only slowly reintroduce those foods that you have been avoiding. And take note as to how you feel as you do return to your old habits. You may find that you do not digest some things as easily as before. Such signs offer a great opportunity for you to change your eating habits for the better.

Other Ways to Detoxify Naturally

There are a number of natural healing methods that can support your body in its cleansing efforts. Here are some tried-and-true methods for removing wastes and detoxifying.

Medicinal Plants

The green pharmacy offers a number of herbs and other plant allies that can help free the body of metabolic wastes and poisons. Some of these beneficial flora are discussed below. Many of these healing plants have long been used in what are known as *spring tonics*. This name derives from the fact that the folk healing traditions of many cultures, both European and otherwise, have long recognized that these plants are best used after the cold winter months, when the body is ready to cleanse.

Preparing Teas

Teas are the best known and most common way to make use of the healing powers of plants. A tea can be made from just one plant or from a mixture of different plants. Preparing and using teas is a simple and uncomplicated process. Many teas can also be used as part of a longer cure. One basic rule for preparing tea is to allow the roots and more solid plant parts, if they are used, to soak in cold water before bringing them to a boil. In contrast, to prevent the loss of their valuable constituents, do not boil flowers and leaves. Rather, pour boiling water over the flowers and leaves and allow them to steep in the water as it cools.

Here are basic recipes you can use to prepare a tea out of any of the cleansing and detoxifying medicinal plants discussed below:

- **For flowers and leaves:** Bring one cup (a quarter liter) of water to a boil; pour it over one teaspoonful of the dried herbs and allow it to steep for ten minutes. Strain the tea through a sieve.

- **For roots or bark:** Add one teaspoonful of the solid plant material per one cup (a quarter liter) of cold water and then bring this to a boil. You may want to make several cups of decoction (boiled tea) at a time. Allow the plant material to continue boiling for eight minutes, then remove the tea from the heat source. Strain the tea through a sieve.

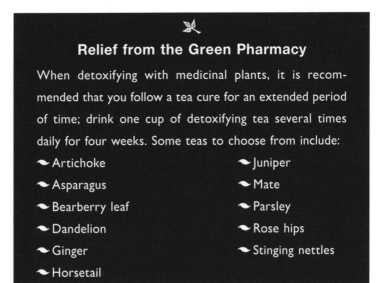

Relief from the Green Pharmacy

When detoxifying with medicinal plants, it is recommended that you follow a tea cure for an extended period of time; drink one cup of detoxifying tea several times daily for four weeks. Some teas to choose from include:

- Artichoke
- Asparagus
- Bearberry leaf
- Dandelion
- Ginger
- Horsetail
- Juniper
- Mate
- Parsley
- Rose hips
- Stinging nettles

On the following pages you will learn more about some of the medicinal plants recommended for detoxification. In addition to their cleansing properties, these plants may also exert other beneficial effects.

Artichoke (*Cynara scolymus*)

The artichoke is a flower—actually, a type of thistle—that is a feast for the eye as well as the palate; with the pretty violet flower it develops, it can be used as a centerpiece on the dining room table or placed in a vase as part of a decorative arrangement. Commonly eaten as a delicious culinary treat, the leaves of the flower of *Cynara scolymus* have tremendous healing benefits when used for medicinal purposes.

Since antiquity, artichokes have been used to support the functioning of the liver and gallbladder and for cleansing and detoxification. In addition, artichokes also promote digestion, regulate blood lipid levels, stimulate the metabolism, and have antioxidative effects that provide protection from the harmful effects of free radicals. Today, ancient knowledge about the effects of the leaves of *Cynara scolymus* has received substantiation from a growing number of scientific studies.* These have confirmed the positive effects that artichokes have in removing metabolic waste and detoxifying the body. Many health food and other stores now offer preparations that include artichoke, including pressed juices, tinctures, and leaf extracts.

Ginger (*Zingiber officinale*)

Although ginger cannot do everything, it can do quite a lot. This is a plant well worth knowing about, for the root of the ginger plant contains a number of substances known to improve health. Traditional Chinese medicine has long counted it among the "royal plants." But the wrinkled, antler-like roots have also been treasured in other countries for centuries.

Ginger owes its potent effects to its high content of

---

*A few of the many studies conducted on the health benefits of *Cynara scolymus:* D'Antuono, A. Garbetta, V. Linsalata, et al., "Polyphenols from artichoke heads (*Cynara cardunculus* (L.) subsp. *scolymus* Hayek): In vitro bio-accessibility, intestinal uptake and bioavailability," *Food and Function* 6, no. 4 (2015): doi:10.1039/c5fo00137d; R. Punzi, A. Paradiso, C. Fasciano, et al., "Phenols and antioxidant activity in vitro and in vivo of aqueous extracts obtained by ultrasound-assisted extraction from artichoke by-products," *Natural Product Communications* 9, no. 9 (2014): 1315–18; A. Villiger, F. Sala, A. Suter, and V. Butterweck, "In vitro inhibitory potential of *Cynara scolymus, Silybum marianum, Taraxacum officinale,* and *Peumus boldus* on key enzymes relevant to metabolic syndrome," *Phytomedicine* 22, no. 1 (2015): 138–44; and N. Xia, A. Pautz, U. Wollscheid, et al., "Artichoke, cynarin and cyanidin downregulate the expression of inducible nitric oxide synthase in human coronary smooth muscle cells," *Molecules* 19, no. 3 (2014): 3654–68.

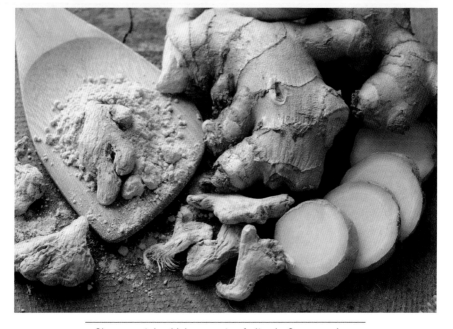

Ginger contains high amounts of vitamin C, magnesium, iron, calcium, potassium, sodium, and phosphorus. It also has potent antibacterial properties.

essential oils and bitter agents. These are good for removing metabolic wastes and other toxins, as well as for lowering elevated LDL cholesterol levels and reducing high blood pressure. These substances also promote circulation, have antioxidative effects, reduce flatulence, aid digestion, and strengthen the heart and immune systems. Ginger also has antiseptic, anti-inflammatory, and analgesic effects. Taken as a tea, tincture, or powder, ginger can help alleviate nausea.

Ginger juice is an excellent tonic that stimulates the appetite and digestion. To make ginger juice, grate a piece of peeled root and squeeze the gratings through a piece of cheesecloth. To make ginger tea, pour boiling water over a gram (one teaspoon is approximately three grams) of pulverized ginger. Allow the tea to steep for five minutes and then strain. Ginger tea should be drunk before eating.

Parsley (*Petroselinum crispum*)

Who would have thought that one of our most popular culinary herbs would contain so many health-promoting substances? Yet this is the reason why parsley has long been held in high esteem outside the kitchen as well as in it. For one thing, parsley is quite rich in vitamins and minerals. Twenty grams (0.71 ounces) of chopped parsley is enough to cover two-thirds of our daily vitamin C requirement. The minerals found in parsley include iron, potassium, and calcium; also present are folic acid and niacin. The essential oils found in parsley, myristicin and apiol, have diuretic and antispasmodic properties. Myristicin, which is also found in nutmeg, has mild psychoactive and inebriating effects; apiol stimulates the digestive processes and menstruation and also has mild germicidal properties. Since parsley dilates the blood vessels of the kidneys, it facilitates kidney function; when combined with potassium, this can have pronounced diuretic effects.

In addition to its usefulness in detoxifying, the properties of parsley also make it well suited for stimulating the digestion and as a general tonic. Parsley thus gently affects the excretion of toxins and metabolic wastes via the kidneys without causing the body to lose high quantities of important minerals.

To undertake a "parsley cure": eat several stalks of fresh parsley (best grown in your own window box or kitchen garden) daily for three weeks while also drinking four cups of parsley tea daily. After adhering to this regimen for three weeks, you should then completely abstain from parsley for eight weeks. Avoid using it even as a garnish or cooking spice during this time.

Parsley Tea

Place approximately one-quarter cup of fresh parsley in an infusion basket. Put the basket into a cup or teapot and pour one cup of filtered boiling water over it. Allow to steep for five to seven minutes. Remove the basket to remove the parsley. You may want to sweeten with honey or stevia and add a fresh bit of lemon juice to enhance the flavor. Enjoy!

Parsley Facial Toner

Wash a handful of fresh parsley, place in a mason jar, and add 100 ml (3 ½ ounces) of 70 percent alcohol. Close tightly and allow to sit for one to two weeks. Use a paper filter to remove the solid material, and then dilute with 300 ml (10 ounces) distilled water. This toner is an excellent supplement for daily use in cleaning the oil from your facial skin.

Parsley also has analgesic, antiseptic, and anti-inflammatory properties. And last but not least, parsley makes an excellent agent for cleaning oily and blemished skin.

Stinging Nettles (*Urtica dioica, Urtica urens*)

Stinging nettles have a long history of use as a spice and vegetable as well a medicinal plant with detoxifying effects that stimulates our metabolic processes. Studies have shown that stinging nettles help inhibit the enzyme aromatase, which can inhibit both the conversion of the male sex hormone testosterone to dihydrotestosterone in the prostate and the

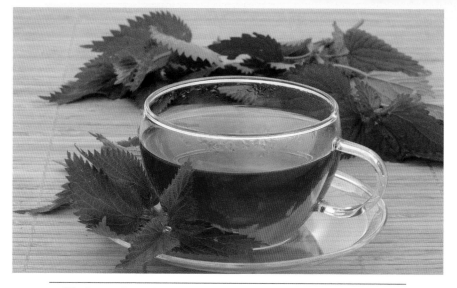
Stinging nettle tea has diuretic, anti-inflammatory, blood-building, and blood-purifying effects. It also stimulates the metabolism.

synthesis of what is sometimes referred to as prostatic growth factor (PGF).*

Stinging nettles are a proven ingredient of tea mixtures used to treat gout, rheumatism, and liver and gallbladder ailments and as a diuretic, for expelling excess fluid from the body. Both stinging nettle teas as well as various preparations of stinging nettle extracts are available from health food stores and other sources. Stinging nettle juice is well suited for spring cures and for weight loss programs.

Spring Tonics for Purification

Spring tonics are old-fashioned folk remedies traditionally used in the springtime, when the herbs used in these tonics are

---

*R. W. Hartmann, M. Mark, and F. Soldati, "Inhibition of 5 α-reductase and aromatase by PHL-00801 (Prostatonin®), a combination of PY102 (*Pygeum africanum*) and UR102 (*Urtica dioica*) extracts," *Phytomedicine* 3, no. 2 (1996): 121–28; and D. Gansser and G. Spiteller, "Aromatase inhibitors from *Urtica dioica* roots," *Planta Medica* 61, no. 2 (1995): 138–40.

usually plentiful. Said to help revive your body after winter's sluggish eating and exercise habits, these herbs are bitter and refreshing. Here are directions for a few spring tonics.

Asparagus Cure

Because asparagus is one of the most exquisite culinary delicacies known, most people do not think of using it for detoxifying. Not only is asparagus low in calories, but its high mineral and vitamin content make it extremely healthy, and it is also a useful diuretic. When our grandmothers wanted to concoct a simple and effective spring tonic, they simply drank the water in which asparagus had been cooked (by itself or mixed with other liquids) or added mashed potatoes and sour cream to the asparagus water to make a soup. To carry out an asparagus cure, however, you should not only drink asparagus water

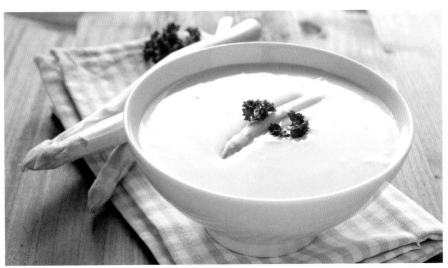

Due to its high potassium content, asparagus can be used as a diuretic. It also contains sodium, calcium, magnesium, phosphorus, iron, and a variety of vitamins.

but also eat at least one pound of fresh asparagus daily for two weeks, prepared according to taste.

Dandelion Cure

Dandelion is an outstanding plant for purging wastes and excess water from the body. This makes it wonderfully suited for a spring tonic. It can be consumed as a salad or in liquid form. To make a salad, pick the tart young leaves, wash them well, and serve chopped and prepared to taste. Adding a bit of yogurt or sweet cream to your salad dressing will help temper the dandelion's slightly bitter taste. You should also take one tablespoon of dandelion juice daily before meals for four weeks. You can make dandelion juice by pressing the leaves and roots yourself, but the process is time-consuming. An easier method is to purchase bottled dandelion juice from a health food store.

Plantain Leaf Juice

In folk medicine, plantain leaf (from *Plantago lanceolata,* not to be confused with the plantain banana) is regarded as a valuable detoxifying agent as well as beneficial for treatment of disorders of the respiratory tract and skin and for insect bites and infections. To make plantain leaf juice, collect four handfuls of plantain leaves and put them through a juicer. Take one teaspoon of the fresh-pressed leaf juice three times daily for two weeks.

Stinging Nettle Cure

Stinging nettles, mentioned earlier in this chapter, are another medicinal plant with purifying properties. Teas made with stinging nettles are a very popular folk remedy. Stinging nettle tea stimulates kidney function, which helps to both promote urination and treats urinary retention.

To prepare stinging nettle tea, boil a cup of water, then place a teaspoon of fresh or dried stinging nettles in the water (do not boil). Allow the tea to steep for a few minutes, and then strain out the leaves using a sieve. Drink four cups of stinging nettle tea daily for three weeks for the "cure." Afterward take a break for approximately two months so that the body does not become too accustomed to the herb, thereby diminishing its detoxifying effects.

Homeopathic Medicine

The compendious materia medica of homeopathic medicine contains many agents that promote the elimination of metabolic wastes and toxins. The great effectiveness of homeopathic medicines in helping to maintain and restore health and in the treatment of numerous ailments is astonishing. These agents function on the basis of the seemingly paradoxical principle that the more diluted a substance is, the more effective it will be.

To manufacture homeopathic preparations, the starting substance, called a *mother tincture,* is successively diluted. In the first stage of this potentiation process, one part of the starting substance is mixed with nine parts lactose or alcohol. The resulting mixture, referred to as *D1* (D referring to "decimal"), contains 10 percent (or a 1:10 ratio) of the mother tincture. This process can be repeated as often as needed to achieve the desired potency. For example, with D6, or the sixth decimal potency, the preceding dilutions have been repeatedly diluted at a 1:10 ratio. The six successive dilutions mean that a D6 potency contains a millionth of the original mother tincture. At D12, the ratio is one molecule of mineral salt to one trillion lactose molecules. At high dilutions of C30 or D30 and above, the scale of dilution is so great that it is as if an aspirin tablet had been dissolved in the Atlantic Ocean; not a single molecule of the mother tincture can be detected in these dilutions. Thus, homeopathy relies not on physical matter but on the healing energy that is carried from the mother tincture to the dilution. In fact, the more diluted the mixture is, the more unadulterated is this healing energy.

Homeopathy works on the principle that the information about the mother tincture's effects is stored in the homeopathic preparation in an energetic form. This is the principle that the German physician Samuel Hahnemann, the founder of homeopathy, postulated some two centuries ago, and it is still followed by homeopathic practitioners today.

Homeopathic "Cleansing"

Homeopathic medicines stimulate the body's self-regulating systems, thereby giving the excretory organs both the crucial impulse to increase their activity and the energy they require to do this. However, it should be noted that treating oneself violates the rules of classical homeopathy, for its focus is to determine the factors that have hindered a person's healing powers and thus led to the appearance of the symptoms of illness. In most cases the person is unaware of these factors. It is the task of the experienced homeopathic practitioner to uncover these hidden factors.

There are, nevertheless, a few homeopathic preparations

that you may use on yourself to cleanse your body of harmful substances and waste products, and some of these are listed below. These preparations are available without a prescription, and different manufacturers may produce them in either a small globule form or a tablet. When you take homeopathics, it is important to reduce or eliminate your intake of caffeine and certain other substances such as alcohol and essential oils, especially menthol and camphor, because they can impair the effects of homeopathic remedies.

Be aware that homeopathic medicine considers it normal for one's symptoms to temporarily worsen after the beginning of treatment. This period of initial worsening may be a reaction of the body and is an indication that the body's self-healing powers have been activated. For this reason, this temporary worsening is taken as a positive sign.

NUX VOMICA D6

NUX VOMICA, also known as the "poison nut," stimulates the intestines and kidneys. It also alleviates digestive complaints, flatulence, and feelings of satiety. Take five globules (or tablets) three times daily.

SULFUR D12

SULFUR induces a deep body cleansing. It has potent detoxifying effects on the connective tissues and mucous membranes and helps expel such harmful substances as environmental toxins. This is the reason why SULFUR is administered in homeopathy when other homeopathic remedies have lost their effectiveness because the body is overloaded with waste products and toxins. Take three globules (or tablets) of SULFUR three times daily.

GELSEMIUM D6

When detoxifying, you can sometimes experience short-term headaches and dizzy spells. Yellow jasmine—the plant name for the homeopathic GELSEMIUM—will help these ailments quickly pass. Take five globules (or tablets) three times daily.

PULSATILLA D6

The small pasqueflower works its detoxifying effects primarily on the mucous membranes, especially those of the stomach and digestive tract and the respiratory passages. It is particularly recommended for clearing out the harmful substances that can accumulate from using pharmaceutical drugs. Take three globules (or tablets) of PULSATILLA three times daily.

ARSENICUM ALBUM D12

In keeping with the homeopathic principle that "like cures like," the very same substance that cost many people their lives in the form of poison (it was once popular as such) is used in homeopathy as a kind of universal antidote for detoxifying. ARSENICUM ALBUM has profound effects on the tissues and all of our organs. It is particularly well suited for ridding the body of excessive accumulations of wastes due to long-term nutritional sins. Take two globules (or tablets) of ARSENICUM ALBUM three times daily.

BERBERIS VULGARIS D6

Barberry intensively stimulates the gallbladder, liver, and kidneys. In this respect it is ideal for purging the body of everything that is harmful and unnecessary. Take five globules (or tablets) of BERBERIS VULGARIS three times daily.

❧

Hahnemann's Revolutionary Therapy

Dr. Christian Friedrich Samuel Hahnemann (1755–1843), a physician from Meissen, Germany, established the fundamentals of homeopathy. Even today, the entire field of homeopathy is based on his medical insights. Homeopathy grew out of a 1790 experiment Hahnemann conducted on the bark of the cinchona (*Cinchona pubescens*) or quina tree. This provided him with the impulse to develop this healing method, which is based on an innovative understanding of health and illness. The cinchona experiment demonstrated that a substance that can produce certain symptoms in a healthy person can also be used to treat those very same symptoms. His work ultimately led Hahnemann to set down the basic rule of homeopathy, the similarity principle *similia similibus curantus*, "like cures like." This revolutionary insight turned the assump-

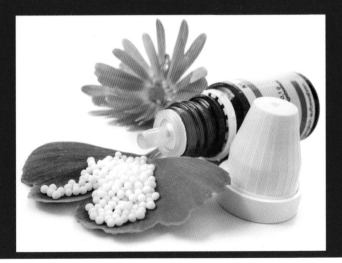

tions on which medicine had been based up until that time on their head. Until Hahnemann's time, physicians were convinced that to treat an illness it was necessary to alleviate its symptoms. In contrast, the homeopathic doctrine prescribes the use of substances derived from animal, plant, and mineral sources that provoke those symptoms. These substances are administered in a substantially diluted and shaken form (potency). In other words, the medicinal preparations that are administered are primarily intended not to fight off an illness and its symptoms but to increase the body's natural defenses and activate its innate self-healing powers. In this manner, the body is supported in its efforts to overcome the illness.

Schüssler Salts

The German physician Dr. Wilhelm Heinrich Schüssler (1821–1889) pioneered a range of homeopathic cell salts, the use of which remains enormously popular today. There are many reasons why his healing method has not been forgotten since his time. Because they nourish the cells, Schüssler's cell salts can have a profound impact on our health. They strengthen the organism and protect its functions without causing any side effects or interacting with other substances. Schüssler salts are also well suited for detoxifying and cleansing the body.

Healthy Cells, Healthy Body

Dr. Schüssler asserted that the health of our cells is the basis for the well-being of the entire organism. According to his theory, illness is the result of a disturbance in cellular functioning. Because it was already known in his time that minerals play a central role in cellular functions, Schüssler concluded that a person can only remain healthy when all of the necessary minerals are present in the proper amounts and the proper proportions to one another. If this is not the case, the cells' metabolism can become unbalanced. Such disturbances in the body's cellular metabolism can lead to disturbances in health, but if the cells can be provided with the proper amounts of the missing minerals, then those functions that have been disrupted by these deficiencies can be rectified and the cell functions restored. Dr. Schüssler's treatment method, which he called *biochemical therapy* (*bios,* "life," and *chemie,* "the study of the properties and composition of substances"), is based on this insight. Accordingly, the homeopathic cell salts that Schüssler developed are also referred to as the "salts of life."

Before he could achieve his final breakthrough, however, Schüssler had to overcome a crucial hurdle. He already knew that pure minerals are not easily absorbed by the body. While sufficient quantities of these minerals might be present in our diet, our various cells cannot absorb them all to the same degree. How could he ensure that each individual cell would receive the amount that it required in order to function properly? Schüssler, who was also a homeopath, soon found his answer. To achieve the optimal absorption of these mineral substances—in other words, to ensure their "bioavailability"—he turned to a method derived from homeopathy. He diluted the mineral salts substantially so that they could more quickly arrive where they were needed: by immediately passing from the mucous membranes in the mouth, throat, and esophagus into the blood, and from there, traveling directly to the cells. By means of this so-called potentiation, the increasingly fine digestion of the mother substance serves to enhance its effects. The results of Dr. Schüssler's groundbreaking work, Schüssler salts, are now widely available in the United States, in health food and vitamin stores and at online retailers.

Schüssler's Homeopathic Roots

The founder of homeopathy, Samuel Hahnemann, taught that illnesses can be cured with minute amounts of those very same substances that evoke the symptoms of illness. This is the principle of homeopathy, "like cures like." However, even though the treatment methods of both Schüssler salts and homeopathy are based on the same technique of potentiation, the two do differ somewhat. Schüssler, who practiced homeopathic medicine, said that strictly speaking, his healing methods were not precisely the same as the "like cures like" principle underlying homeopathic methods, but rather were based on the "physiological-chemical operations" that occur in the body. In other words, Schüssler did not follow the homeopathic principle of similarity when selecting the compounds he would prescribe. Therefore, when using the salts of life, the effects do not need to match the symptoms of the illness that is being treated.

How the Salts of Life Work

Schüssler salts exert a regulatory effect on cellular metabolism. In contrast to typical mineral preparations, the salts of

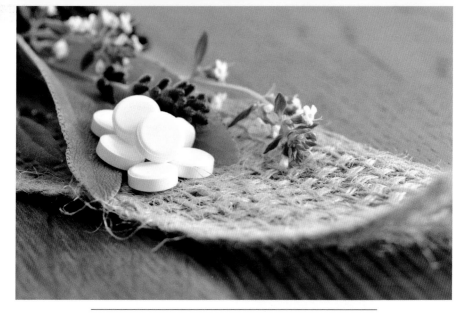

Schüssler salts mobilize the self-healing powers of the body
by regulating the mineral balance on the cellular level.

life are aimed not at increasing the amounts of deficient minerals, but at helping the cells make optimal use of the minerals present in the diet. This difference is achieved as a result of how the salts are prepared. Because of their potentiation, the effects of Schüssler salts differ from those of less refined materials: they provide the cells with information that enables them to better utilize the available nutrients, thereby providing them with the impulse to return to equilibrium. This enables the body's own abilities to heal itself to be stabilized from the ground up. Another way this can be seen is through the markedly good detoxification effects produced by many of the Schüssler salts.

How to Use Schüssler Salts

To achieve the full benefits of Schüssler salts, you should consider several things:

- Schüssler salts are to be not swallowed but slowly dissolved under the tongue, the same as with taking a homeopathic remedy. This is a fundamental principle of this method, as the effects are said to begin as the finely crushed medicinal preparation is absorbed sublingually, through the mouth's mucous membranes. Consequently, the slow dissolution of the material under the tongue is part of the healing process.

- Do not ingest the salts with a meal. The rule of thumb is to take them thirty minutes before or one hour after a meal.

- Coffee, black tea, peppermint, cocoa, essential oils, and artificial sugars can affect the uptake of Schüssler salts, just as they can homeopathics. For this reason you should abstain from using them directly before or after you use the salts.

- When you're using the salts for detoxifying, take two tablets three times daily.

The Twelve Functional Substances

Dr. Schüssler continuously refined his treatment methods and ultimately developed a therapy using only twelve carefully selected mineral salts. He referred to these as "functional substances," because each of these twelve remedies supports specific functions in the cells, tissues, and organs. Schüssler recommended using the majority of these functional substances at a potency of D6. The exceptions are salts no. 1, 3, and 11, which are administered at a potency of D12.

The Standard Potencies
of the Twelve Salts

➤ No. 1 CALCIUM FLUORATUM	D12
➤ No. 2 CALCIUM PHOSPHORICUM	D6
➤ No. 3 FERRUM PHOSPHORICUM	D12
➤ No. 4 KALIUM CHLORATUM	D6
➤ No. 5 KALIUM PHOSPHORICUM	D6
➤ No. 6 KALIUM SULFURICUM	D6
➤ No. 7 MAGNESIUM PHOSPHORICUM	D6
➤ No. 8 NATRIUM CHLORATUM	D6
➤ No. 9 NATRIUM PHOSPHORICUM	D6
➤ No. 10 NATRIUM SULFURICUM	D6
➤ No. 11 SILICEA	D12
➤ No. 12 CALCIUM SULFURICUM	D6

Schüssler Salts for Detoxifying and Cleansing

The following lists those salts of life that provide the most effective support for detoxifying and cleansing the body of metabolic wastes and other toxins. You may decide to use just one or two of the four salts presented here. Take two tablets of each of the salts you will be using three times daily. It is best to take the Schüssler salts for four to six weeks as part of a therapeutic cure.

Salt No. 6—KALIUM SULFURICUM

The sixth of the functional substances is the salt for metabolism and detoxification and for the liver, skin, and mucous membranes. It activates the cellular metabolism and functions of the liver, one of our most important excretory and detoxifi-

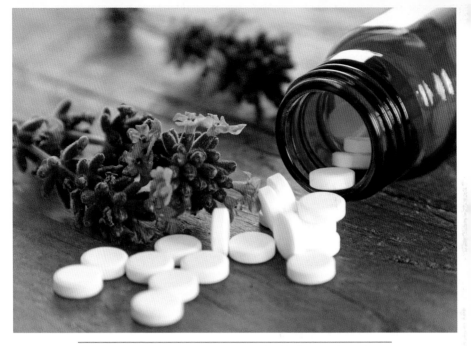

To manufacture his mineral salts, Dr. Schüssler adopted homeopathic ideas about dilution and potentiation.

cation organs. KALIUM SULFURICUM also stimulates protein metabolism, which leads to the increased excretion of metabolic wastes and toxins. In addition, it can help with rheumatic ankle pains and slow digestion.

Salt No. 9—NATRIUM PHOSPHORICUM

This is the salt used to treat the metabolic and lymphatic systems and to regulate the acid-alkaline balance. This salt carries out a number of tasks involved in the complex processes of metabolism, especially in getting rid of metabolic wastes. Salt no. 9 is essential for the excretion of excess acids, which are produced by every metabolic process. It also helps regulate fat metabolism. NATRIUM PHOSPHORICUM also stimulates kidney functioning and is useful in the treatment of acne, inflammations, metabolic disturbances, and digestive difficulties.

Salt No. 10—NATRIUM SULFURICUM

This has been called the salt for excretion, detoxification, and digestion. It is used to aid the body in removing excess metabolic waste and poisons in the fastest way possible. Because of this activity, this salt is found less frequently in the cells than in the tissue fluids, the very site where the body deposits most of the wastes it produces as it metabolizes and breaks down the chemicals within. In light of these effects, NATRIUM SULFURICUM is especially effective on the excretory organs: the liver, kidneys, and bladder. The gallbladder and stomach are also powerfully supported by this salt. NATRIUM SULFURICUM also works well in cases of ailments caused by meals that are overly rich or fatty, and it addresses flatulence, diarrhea, and other digestive disturbances as well.

Salt No. 11—SILICEA

As the salt for the skin, hair, nails, connective tissues, and nerves, SILICEA is the "cosmetic of biochemical therapy." This is primarily due to the fact that SILICEA promotes the excretion of excess wastes and metabolic poisons from the connective tissues. This leads to a tightening and firming of the connective tissue and the elimination of cellulite on the buttocks and thighs. SILICEA also helps prevent varicose veins and arthrosclerosis and aids in healing wounds and other injuries.

Fasting

Whether done to facilitate mental contemplation, as a religious ritual, or as a type of sacrifice, the practice of temporarily discontinuing the intake of food has a long tradition in human history and in cultures throughout the world. Yet the most important reason for fasting has been and continues to be the fact that it is an effective means to care for our health, because fasting relieves the entire organism, refreshes the intestinal flora from top to bottom, strengthens the immune system, and helps lower high blood pressure. It also has detoxifying and cleansing effects. Finally, interrupting the otherwise constant supply of food gives the body and its cleaning crew a long-needed opportunity to clean things up and recover from their exertions. This provides long-lasting effects and has helped many people change their unhealthy eating habits. This is one reason why people often refer to such practices as "healing fasts."

Fasting also helps clean out our emotional closets, as our normal activities create psychological as well as physical waste products. Fasting can help rid us of both. In short, after completing a fast, we feel as if we have been reborn, both physically and emotionally.

The term *fast* encompasses a wide variety of practices. In the current context, we can only describe the most important principles on which this traditional method of healing rests.

Fasting Correctly

A fast should generally be undertaken for one week. Those who still feel fit when this time has passed may stretch this to ten days. You should break your fast by slowly starting to eat again. Apart from drinking weak black, green, or white tea, it is best to abstain from coffee, alcohol, and all other such substances while you are fasting.

When Should You Refrain from Fasting?

In principle, anyone who is healthy and fit and who has the willpower to persevere can undertake a fast of several days. However, there are situations and ailments for which fasting is not advised:

- If you are suffering from some type of depressive disorder
- If you are underweight
- If you are facing great challenges in your professional or personal life
- When dealing with severe physical and mental exhaustion
- When convalescing from an illness or after an accident or operation
- If you have an overactive thyroid
- If you have a stomach ulcer or gastritis
- If you are pregnant
- If you are lactating
- If you are suffering from an eating disorder like anorexia or bulimia

On the Day before Your Fast

On the day before you actually begin your fast you should try to relax and prepare yourself for the food-free days to come. You should also prepare your body by eating nothing but fresh fruit on this day.

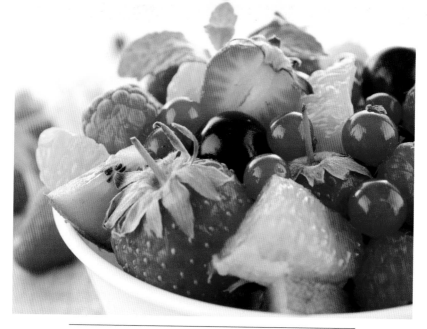

Fresh fruit, especially in summer when there is a plentiful
supply of fresh berries and fruits available, is the ideal food
to eat in preparation for a fast.

What You Will Need to Fast

- An enema device or about an ounce (30 grams)
  of Glauber's salt (sodium sulfate or a similar
  preparation)
- Mineral water, herbal teas, fruit juices, vegetable
  broths, and buttermilk (as desired)

As needed:

- Hot water bottle
- Massage brush or loofah
- Massage oil
- Lemon juice
- Healing clay (for internal use)

First Day

Your first day of fasting begins with a thorough cleansing of your digestive system. Dissolve about an ounce and a half (forty grams) of Glauber's salt or a similar preparation in a little over two cups (one-half liter) of water, add a few squirts of lemon juice, and drink the mixture. After you have ingested all of it, drink sufficient water or herbal tea to get rid of the salt taste. A profound colonic cleansing should take place over the next one to three hours.* Once you have ingested Glauber's salt, you should absolutely plan on staying at home, as the urge to evacuate will hit you spontaneously and in quick succession. Some people prefer an enema, which cleans the colon in a gentler manner than Glauber's salt.

For the rest of this first day relax, read, sleep, or take a walk. Be sure to avoid any excessive activities, including hot baths, because these can place a great burden on your circulatory system.

Second Day

Feelings of hunger often occur during the second day of the fast. If this happens, drink a glass of mineral water or a few sips of buttermilk. If that does not help, administer a second enema to empty your bowels. If you have mild sensations of dizziness (a completely normal occurrence during a fast), take a walk in the fresh air or lie down and refresh yourself with cold water. Your body is now in a transition phase in which it is exhausting its own reserves. Your blood pressure may fall

---

*Because Glauber's salt may irritate the membranes of the colon, persons with sensitive colons or other digestive issues should not use it and should substitute some other method, such as an enema.

during this time. This is why it is generally recommended that people who are fasting avoid overly exerting themselves and steer clear of physical and mental stress.

Third Day

Your body has now made the transition. Usually feelings of hunger and circulatory problems are no longer an issue. You can engage in some gentle activities such as yoga, going for a walk, or taking a relaxed swim, but be careful not to overdo it. Only pursue these activities as long as you enjoy them and you continue to feel good.

The Following Days

The remainder of your fast will most likely pass without problems. Be sure to drink lots of fluids—at least eight cups a day. The best things to drink are mineral water, fruit juice (unsweetened and diluted with water), herbal and fruit teas, and vegetable-based broths. Avoid getting up too quickly in the morning. Instead, sit for a moment at the edge of your bed and dry-brush yourself with a massage brush or a loofah glove (see the box on the following page). This will help stabilize your circulation, making you fit to begin your day. If your sense of taste seems off, try gargling with healing clay (for internal use) or chew some parsley or chives.

Breaking Your Fast

Take it slowly when you begin eating again. Raw fruits are easy to digest and a good place to begin. Unsweetened yogurt (or another living cultured milk product) is also a good fast breaker. As you break your fast, eat frequent small meals and stop eating as soon as you begin to feel full. Keep your meals very simple and easy to digest at first. In the days following the fast you can gradually add to your meals, incorporating raw lettuce and spinach, cooked vegetables and vegetable soups, other raw vegetables, well-cooked grains and beans, nuts and eggs, noncultured dairy products, and finally meat.

Brush Away Toxins

Dry-brushing the skin is a proven method of detoxification, as the skin is a vital part of the human excretory system. Brushing the skin stimulates the skin's circulation and metabolic processes. This aids in transporting toxins out of organs and in freeing the skin of dead cells. The tissues tighten and the skin becomes better able to absorb skin creams or oils. A dry-brushing massage will leave you feeling physically and emotionally refreshed, relaxed, and ready for the day. For those who have difficulty getting started in the morning, there are few things that are more helpful than dry brushing. For all of these reasons, dry brushing should not be "saved" until you reach a point where illness forces you to purge metabolic wastes and toxins; rather, make it a part of your regular body-care regimen.

All that is needed is a massage brush made of natural fibers with a loop or handle. A sisal glove or mitt is also suitable for this purpose. Such a brush or mitt is available at most health food markets. Here's how you do it:

➤ Begin by brushing, using small, circular motions, the instep of your right foot, then the sole of your foot, and then work your way up to your calf and upward to the right side of your buttocks. Repeat the process from the top of your foot to your hip joint on the front of your leg.

➤ Now work on your left side, beginning with the left instep, sole, and calf and ending with your left buttock. Then repeat on the front of your left leg.

➤ When brushing your upper body, begin with the back of your right hand, then work your way along the upper side of your arm toward your shoulder. Repeat the process along the underside of your arm, starting with your palm and working your way up. Follow the same procedure on your left arm.

➤ Next, brush your chest, working in straight lines from the periphery toward your sternum. Brush the stomach in a clockwise direction, and brush your neck by working from the jaw down toward your shoulders. Finish by brushing your back.

Avoid dry-brushing any areas of the skin that are damaged, that exhibit psoriasis, or that have acne. You should avoid dry brushing altogether if you have an overactive thyroid. You should also refrain from dry-brushing any areas affected by inflamed varicose veins.

Colon Cleansing

Healers have long known that "all evil dwells in the intestine." For this reason, a regular cleansing of this important organ can help to both maintain and restore health. Colon cleansing is the best and most efficient means of freeing the colon of all harmful materials and helping it maintain the proper balance of bacterial flora. When it comes to colon cleansing, there are several methods to choose from. Here are three of the most common:

Colon Hydrotherapy

Strictly speaking, this method is the modern version of an enema. However, it is carried out by a professionally trained therapist using a specialized device that delivers warm, filtered water through the anus and into the colon. This provides a gentle but nevertheless intensive cleansing. Throughout the treatment you lie relaxed on your back on a bed or lounge. During a colon hydrotherapy session (also known as *colonic irrigation*), the practitioner will usually gently massage your belly to both increase the effects and increase your comfort. Colon hydrotherapy currently enjoys great popularity in the United States, and practitioners are to be found in most major cities and many smaller cities.

Glauber's Salt

This natural laxative consists primarily of sodium sulfate. Glauber's salt is available in drugstores and from other sources (although it may be sold under another name). If you intend to use this to perform a colon cleansing it is imperative that you schedule the time at which you will ingest the salt so that you do not have any important appointments in the hours that follow and that you are able to remain near a toilet. Once the effects of the salt make themselves known, you will need to act immediately. (See the previous section on fasting, the first day, for instructions on preparing and drinking Glauber's salt.)

Enema

Enemas offer another method for cleansing the colon. Enemas have the advantage that you can predict the time at which the colon will empty. If you decide to administer an enema in the evening, then you know that your colon will empty in the next few hours. More information about how to administer an enema can be found in the box below.

Administering an Enema

What used to be a part of your grandma's standard set of household remedies is much less uncomfortable and time-consuming than you may think. So give it a try, and not only because it will help you purge your body of old wastes. An enema serves to thoroughly empty and clean out the colon, helping the entire body to quickly and gently detoxify. You can also turn to the enema to treat many acute illnesses, such as fever, digestive ailments, febrile colds, or persistent headaches.

You will need an enema device (available at pharmacies and drugstores) consisting of an eight-inch-long insertion nozzle, an enema bag (irrigator), and an enema syringe. You will also need some petroleum jelly or similar lubricant. Use preboiled and lukewarm water as the enema fluid.

➤ Fill the enema bag with one liter of lukewarm water and hang this over a door handle or a towel rod in the bathroom. Test by allowing the air to run out of the hose and into the sink or the bathtub.

➤ Now connect the enema nozzle to the end of the enema hose and lubricate the tip with petroleum jelly or other lubricant.

➤ Squat or kneel on the bathroom floor. Use your elbows to support your upper body as you slowly insert the enema nozzle into your anus.

➤ Allow the water to flow evenly into the colon as you

gradually insert the nozzle farther into the colon. Be sure to breath slowly and continuously during the process.

➤ Hold the water in your colon until you feel the urge to eliminate (it will feel like you are ready to have a bowel movement). This usually occurs about five minutes after administering the enema.

Take Care when Cleansing Your Colon!

➤ Every method of cleansing the colon results in a loss of fluids. Be sure to balance this out by drinking lots of fluids. Mineral water, unsweetened herbal teas, and diluted and unsweetened fruit and vegetable juices are ideal.

➤ After cleansing the colon, it is important to restore the flora (bacteria) of the colon. This can be achieved using preparations containing high concentrations of *Lactobacillus acidophilus.* These are commonly available at health food stores. You can also support the restoration of healthy digestive flora by consuming products rich in probiotics, such as yogurt, kefir, buttermilk, fresh sauerkraut, and kombucha.

Bathe Your Body's Wastes Away

A lovely way to detoxify that complements all the methods mentioned in this book is to literally bathe the internal "dirt" right out of your system by bathing in essential oils and sea salt. Such mixtures also tighten the tissues and stimulate the circulation. To prepare a full bath, use approximately four cups of sea salt (the best comes from the Dead Sea). Among the essential oils that can be used to detoxify and remove wastes are fennel, grapefruit, rosemary, juniper, lemon, orange, and cypress oils. Add ten drops of the oil of your choice to your bathwater.

One detoxifying and enjoyable method of bathing from the ayurvedic tradition involves taking a bath in wheat germ. Place two handfuls of wheat germ in a fine-mesh linen bag, which you then hang under the faucet so that the hot water flows through it as it fills your tub. When the tub is full, squeeze the remaining fluid out of the bag and into the water. Be careful not to soak for more than ten to fifteen minutes. Afterward, shower without drying yourself off, and instead air-dry in the warm bathroom.

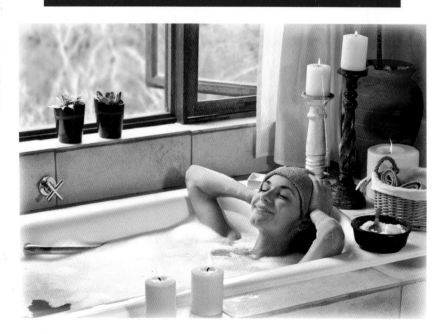

Bibliography

Alphen, Jan van, ed. *Orientalisch Medizin* (Oriental Medicine). Bern, Stuttgart, Vienna: Paul Haupt Verlag, 1997.

Dahlke, Ruediger. *Krankheit als Symbol* (Illness as Symbol). Munich: C. Bertelsmann Verlag, 1996.

Frohn, Birgit. *Die Heilkraft der Olive* (The Healing Powers of the Olive). Murnau: Mankau Verlag. 2012.

———. *Fussreflexzonemassage* (Foot Reflexology Massage). Augsburg: Weltbild Verlag, 1998.

———. *Lexicon der Heilpflanzen* (Encyclopedia of Medicinal Plants). Augsburg: Weltbild Verlag, 2010.

———. *Schmerzfrei durch Fingerdruck* (Pain-Free through Finger Pressure). Augsburg: Weltbild Verlag, 2003.

Frohn, Birgit, and Hans-Heinrich Rhynew. *Heilpflanzen im Ayurveda* (Healing Plants in Ayurveda). Baden and Munich: AT Verlag, 2006.

Frohn, Birgit, Heiner Uber, and Xokonoschletl. *Medizin der Mutter Erde* (Medicine of Mother Earth). Munich: Orbis Verlag, 1996.

Menche, Nicole, ed. *Biologie, Anatomy, Physiologie* (Biology, Anatomy, Physiology). Munich: Urban & Fischer Verlag, 2007.

Wolfram, Katharina. *Die Ölzieh-Kur* (The Oil Pulling Cure). Darmstadt: Schirner Verlag, 2008.

Index

Images

HLPhoto – Fotolia.com (i)

fredredhat – Fotolia.com (vi)

tomasworks – iStockphoto.com (6)

fovito – Fotolia.com (10)

Jacek Chabraszewski – Fotolia.com (13)

arsdigital – Fotolia.com (17)

Henrik5000 – iStockphoto.com (23)

Kurhan – Fotolia.com (25)

Robert Kneschke – Fotolia.com (27)

lu-photo – Fotolia.com (31)

HLPhoto – Fotolia.com (34)

Knut Wiarda – Fotolia.com (37)

Murat Subatli – Fotolia.com (41)

Jeanette Dietl – Fotolia.com (42)

Christian Jung – Fotolia.com (52)

Marina Lohrbach – Fotolia.com (54)

billnoll – iStockphoto.com (58)

Corinna Gissemann – Fotolia.com (64)

alexxx1981 – iStockphoto.com (66)

Riccardo bruni – Fotolia.com (68)

Giuseppe Porzani – Fotolia.com (80)

egal – iStockphoto.com (88)

LianeM – Fotolia.com (91)

CGissemann – Fotolia.com (92)

Alexander Raths – Fotolia.com (98)

tinlinx – Fotolia.com (102)

Kathrin39 – Fotolia.com (105)

M.studio – Fotolia.com (109)

Anna Omelchenko – Fotolia.com (117)